I0435560

BLISSFUL BODY
PAINLESS PATH

From chronic pain to personal power!

By

Maria Bott

www.mariabott.com

TESTIMONIALS

"Working with Maria has been a pleasure and an insightful journey. After suffering with pain for over ten years, she taught me to connect my mind, body, and spirit to significantly improve my overall well-being. Her rich knowledge of anatomy, wise instruction, intelligence and dedication enabled me to regain my health where other methods had failed.

Maria has been a huge blessing in my life, and I am so thankful to have found her."

Gloria C.
Tampa, Florida client

"I have worked with many personal trainers in the past, but Maria's enthusiasm and knowledge is unmatched. While I was not in bad shape or overweight - Maria quickly changed my body by proposing a routine for realignment, agility and balance. With yoga and circuit training and specific breathing techniques, the results have been incredible physically and mentally.

Maria has worked on correcting my body, my strength and my attitude and I have felt the difference. I feel stronger physically as well as mentally with her as my trainer and life coach. She has kept me focused and given me more vitality to focus on my work as well as keeping me more positive throughout the day.

Maria takes her clients on an emotional and physical journey. She has made dramatic changes in my physical appearance, energy levels, strength and stamina and I am grateful to have her in my life."

Jillian A.
Tampa, Florida client

"Maria was recommended to me by my chiropractor to help me stretch and relax muscles in my lower and upper back, so that he could properly adjust my spine. I was having trouble breathing because of muscle patterns that I had formed over my life that constricted my airway.

With Maria's help I have changed many of my muscle patterns enabling me to breathe better, walk better, and feel better overall. In addition, I have gained flexibility and neuromuscular strength. I can squat with ease now. I can use my elliptical machine without cramping.

Maria has truly enhanced my ability to move as well as my endurance in all my activities of daily living."

Miguel C.

Tampa, Florida client

Copyright © 2014, by Maria Bott

DISCLAIMER

The information presented in this book is true and complete to the best of the author's knowledge. This book is an information guide only. It is intended for people seeking relief from chronic pain that is not related to an illness or injury. In no way is this book intended to replace, or to conflict with the advice given to you by your physician. Any lifestyle changes that you make, or decisions regarding your wellbeing, are solely your own responsibility. The information presented here is general, and in no way offers or implies a guarantee. The author and publisher disclaim all liability in connection with the use of this book.

DEDICATION

I dedicate this book to my mother Marjorie Bott. At the age of eighty-eight mum still hangs the washing out on the line to dry, and climbs the stairs in her home with ease. And to my Aunt Aud, who walks to the village hall for line dancing every week. You both inspire me to help myself, and others, to stay active well into the golden years!

This book is also dedicated to the millions of people currently suffering with chronic pain. The solution that will lead to your relief is out there; don't give up until you find it. It's my hope of course that you will find that solution right here, in these pages.

ACKNOWLEDGEMENTS

I acknowledge here the students and clients that have helped me to learn and grow over the years. Through your dedication to improving your health, I have gained a wealth of knowledge and experience.

I also offer praise for the organizations and individuals that I have quoted in this book. Without the benefit and inspiration of your hard work, I wouldn't be the coach that I am today. My heartfelt thanks go out to all of you.

TABLE OF CONTENTS

INTRODUCTION

Experiencing chronic pain at some point in life has become all but expected in society today. I'm not talking about the pain caused by a disease, a broken bone, or a torn ligament. I'm talking about the insidious neck, back, or knee pain that plagues people for weeks, months, and even years!

Sufferers are now numbering in the millions, serving to make this condition appear usual, and to become accepted. Chronic pain is an epidemic that can lower your quality of life, impact your relationships, and lead to dependence on over-the-counter medications.

There are no preferences of sex, culture, age or race when it comes to suffering with chronic pain. The problem is not limited to people who are deconditioned, overweight, or living a sedentary lifestyle either. Athletes, body builders, and yoga and Pilates students are equally at risk of developing a chronic pain chain. The reason for this lies in the basic causes of this chronic condition.

By revealing the origins of the pain chain, and applying the appropriate solutions, relief is the result. No one deserves to be suffering unnecessarily; yet this is exactly what's happening to millions of people today who are living with chronic pain.

MY MOTIVATION

In the early nineteen eighties I was working as a trauma hypnotherapist in England. During that time I witnessed profound events that revealed something to me of the human condition. The clients that I worked with at the time had experienced their traumas months, and in some cases years before coming to see me. Any physical damage done during the accident or attack had long since been resolved.

The sessions were designed to address the emotional blockages and related fears of the client. Yet soon I discovered that the symptoms being presented to me were as much physical, as they were emotional. Victims described to me the anxiety and tension being triggered by memories of their trauma. I actually witnessed a client under hypnosis contort his body into a near impossible position. He was reliving the night of a car crash in which he had been horribly disfigured.

My experience with the powerful mind and body connection continued to expand during my practice of Tai Kwon Do, a Korean marital art. I was the only girl in a class of thirty boys. Standing just five feet four inches tall and weighing one hundred and ten pounds, the idea of breaking wood with my fist at first appeared to be absurd. Quickly I discovered that punching through planks of wood is about skill and focus, not body size or weight.

My teacher taught me to aim beyond the wood; to make the target on the other side of it. He explained that if I aimed at the surface of the wood, my arm would be fully extended and powerless by the time my fist hit the board. Power is found in the focus and determination to pass through all obstacles, and to reach the other side. The obstacle itself is not the target.

This understanding levels the playing field in martial arts. Learning how to break wood taught me that power is realized through knowledge. Knowledge is an aspect of the mind, which manifests as action. I validated this perception at a Tai Kwon Do tournament. My small fist passed through two inches of wood as if it were butter, and using a difficult back-fist strike at that!

A light was now shining brightly for me on the relationship between the mind and the body. I could see clearly how they worked together, and how one would exert influence over the other. I had it all figured out, and at such an early stage in my career. Boy, how quickly that bright light was snuffed out for me one frosty afternoon.

It was 1982, and the Tai Kwon Do examinations at that time were being held in a school gymnasium. The ceilings were high and the windows spanned the entire room. It was freezing the day that I sat in that room with thirty other students waiting to be graded. We all sat crossed legged on the floor, directed to remain still until our names were called out to come forward.

My stomach was churning, as it always does when I'm nervous. Unfortunately for me, I was also born with Palindromic Rheumatism, a rare autoimmune disease. Cold air on my body causes my joints and muscles to become inflamed, and it can be extremely painful. Not being able to 'warm up' took its toll on me even more than it did on the other students.

Four hours dragged by before my name was finally called at the end of the roll. Despite being physically fit, sitting still for so long in that cold room had caused my muscles to contract. When exposed to cold temperatures blood is pulled from external muscles, and directed internally to keep the body warm. I could feel the tension in my muscles. Nonetheless, I did not expect what was about to happen to me.

My stomach was still rumbling, as I positioned myself in front of the easel supporting the wooden boards. I was more concerned about the sparring coming up later on however, than I was about breaking the wood. After all, I'd become quite adept at this point at punching through obstacles.

A hush fell over the gym, as I prepared myself to deliver the blow. In that moment of focus the pain in my body had taken a back seat. With a quick sharp breath I sent my fist flying forwards, aiming at that hidden target behind the stand in front of me.

Looking back at that moment now, I can't recall which pain overwhelmed me first. It could have been the cervical disc as it slipped out of place. Perhaps it was the skin tearing off my knuckles as they dragged across the wood. Needless to say, I failed the grading that day. I also spent the following nine months recovering from the damage to my neck.

My life took a different direction after that incident; I embraced the more gentle science of yoga. Having Palindromic Rheumatism, I decided that practicing Tai Kwon Do wasn't the best choice for my body anymore. Yoga on the other hand is a practice of the 'Citta', which is a Sanskrit word meaning 'the workings of the mind'. Yoga is about understanding that every move your body makes begins as a thought.

That time in my life turned out to be just the beginning of my journey; an exploration into the amazing and intimate connection between the mind and the nervous system. My own suffering spurred me on to find answers to living with chronic pain. I didn't want to learn how to 'manage' my pain - I wanted solutions for relieving it!

My research revealed to me that there's a misconception undermining the comfort of the general population. This misconception is that chronic pain is not only normal, but it's to be expected and accepted as a part of everyday life. There are three common beliefs supporting this misconception:

THE FIRST BELIEF: If the pain is not bad enough to warrant medical attention, then nothing can be done about it.

THE SECOND BELIEF: Your friends have their own pain problems, so you should suffer in silence.

THE THIRD BELIEF: Chronic pain and discomfort automatically come with aging.

From my own experience I can tell you that it's far from natural to be carrying around a chronic pain chain – no matter what age you might be right now. Suffering in silence might make you a martyr, but it won't lead you to finding relief. Last but not least, no matter how dire your situation is today, you can definitely get better as you get older. You too can learn to improve your strength, agility, and overall life experience.

But there's one more important factor that I've realized over the years; the fact is that knowledge alone is not enough. Therefore this book isn't just about physical activity; it's also about mental awareness. It's about delving into what motivates you – or doesn't – to live a personally empowered life. Knowledge only becomes wisdom when it's put to good use.

There's no one simple or effective answer to liberating the population from chronic pain. But there may well be one simple or effective answer that will liberate you. If only one person gains one nugget of information here that leads to relief, that's cause to celebrate. My goal is to end the chronic pain epidemic – one person at a time!

BLISS VERSUS HAPPINESS

Your mind and your body work together as one, so there's no way that you can 'follow your bliss' in life if you're suffering with physical pain. After all, your body is the result of what you're thinking about it. If you don't believe me try to stand up, eat, dance, talk, or do anything at all without thinking about it first.

Self-help material is popping up all over the place on subjects from improving your love life, to creating a powerful workout. The topics are multiplying because people are tired of learning to live with chronic pain. They're demanding answers about the causes, and seeking solutions to the problems. People want their suffering to end.

In my work as a yoga therapist and life coach, I've witnessed in case after case that pain in the mind cannot be separated from pain in the body - and vice versa. What I refer to as 'living in a blissful body', is that state in which pain is no longer experienced as chronic suffering. There's an anecdote in yoga that explains the meaning of 'bliss':

> A man is running across the beach when his attention is suddenly caught up in the beauty of the sunset. In that moment he is fully present and time is standing still for him. His mind is completely quiet, and his body relaxed and at ease. In that one moment of time the man is experiencing bliss.

According to this anecdote, bliss can be explained as:

1. Being fully in the experience of the moment
2. Being free of distracting mind chatter
3. Being completely relaxed and at ease

Bliss cannot be experienced in the mind, or in the body, without simultaneously being experienced in both.

When you're 'being' all of the above without needing a sunset to distract you, you've achieved living in a blissful body. Don't worry if you have a ways to go yet; just desiring to be there is a big step towards success.

The Collins English Dictionary interprets 'bliss' as being 'perfectly happy'. The difference between bliss and happiness though, is that true bliss requires no outside influence. Bliss has no opposite state – you're either experiencing bliss, or you're not. There's no such state as 'unbliss'. You wouldn't lament that being passed over for promotion made you feel unblissful.

Happiness on the other hand does have an opposite state. Outside circumstances influence whether you choose to feel happy, or unhappy. Understanding the difference between bliss and happiness is the beginning of breaking the chronic pain-chain. The following anecdote is an example of this.

John and Jack are the same age, and they both work as a computer analyst. They earn the same wage, and both have a wife and child at home. John finds something to enjoy every day about the work that he's doing, and he feels satisfaction in completing the smallest task. Jack on the other hand complains about his life every day. He bounces back and forth between happiness on the weekends, and feeling unhappy and frustrated the other five days of the week.

Who do you think is more likely to suffer with tension headaches or poor digestion: John or Jack? Understanding the communication between your mind and body is a powerful tool in your wellness bag. Applying that understanding to every thought may seem to be an arduous task at first. Consider though that the alternative is struggling through your day in a body that feels out of control.

I'm sharing here with you in this book what I've learned about body language, and how to correct your movement patterns and bad habits. Remember this however, if you're in chronic pain and believing that you need me, or anyone else to 'fix' you, then you're misunderstanding who holds the power. It's your mind, not mine or anyone else's mind that's in control of your body. You hold the key to finding relief; you just need to learn how to use it.

YOU AND THE USER

As you think, so you move – literally! Take a look at this comparison between how your body moves, and how a computer works:

YOU	A COMPUTER
Your consciousness	The user
Your thoughts	The information from the user
Your nervous system	The software receiving the information
Your body	The hardware housing the software

I know very little about computers. The fact that a computer works the way that it does just amazes me. I understand however, that if I were to take a few classes on the subject it would become a lot less amazing.

The way that 'You' work is beyond amazing to me. The more that I learn about the incredible human being, the more in awe of it I become. I've witnessed people overcome physical limitations through conscious desire, education, and determination. There's no reason why you can't improve your situation in the same way.

COORDINATION

Not being able to chew gum and walk at the same time is hardly a joke. Poor coordination puts you at a greater risk for injury. Clumsiness can impact your confidence, and affect your ability to be at your best in public situations.

Note that damage to the nervous system, certain illnesses, and medications can cause problems with balance and coordination. Consult your physician to rule out any underlying medical causes if you're experiencing these issues.

Three elements are required for well-coordinated movements to take place:

ONE:	Desire to move
TWO:	Awareness of present surroundings
THREE:	Correct muscle pattern contractions

Poor coordination can be caused by an eyesight problem affecting the awareness of surroundings. Sitting close to TV screens, computer monitors, handheld gadgets, and reading materials can take its toll on your eyesight. Eyesight issues can cause poor depth perception, a possible culprit for clumsiness, tripping, and stumbling. If you're having any of these problems, a trip to an optometrist is advised.

Another problem that can disrupt coordination is an imbalance between muscle strength and flexibility. I see this particularly in people who've had a serious injury to a limb in the past. One limb has been favored over the other for a period of weeks, months, or even years. The result is a tendency to knock things over, trip over obstacles, or to stumble to one side.

The original injury has been resolved and therefore disregarded. Even without injury, repetitive sitting or standing to one side can cause the same kind of movement pattern problems. Every person creates unique movement patterns. The answer to restoring balance however, is relatively the same:

1. Stand with your weight evenly distributed on both feet.
2. Sit with both heels touching the ground, or your legs together if in a recliner.

3. Stretch your muscles evenly in distance and duration on both sides.

This may appear to be too obvious, or too simple to be the answer; trust me it's neither. When you stand in line at the bank, the post-office, or the grocery store, are you standing with your weight evenly on both feet?

Every time you sit down at a computer or a dining table, are you sitting with your toes and your heels supported by the ground or a step? Are you making sure that you stretch evenly on both sides of your body every time, without exception?

Over the years I've developed a habit of watching people. I've been pulled out of line at the airport by security more than once because of it! Rarely do I observe *anyone* standing evenly balanced and relaxed for more than a few seconds at a time.

If you find it painful to stand with your weight on both feet, then you may still have an unresolved injury. Talk to your physician about possible testing to find out for sure. There'll be more information about stretching correctly further on in the book.

MIND OVER MATTER

I was having coffee with a friend of mine one morning. She was telling me an exciting story about a past event. Her hands were waving around in the air in tandem to her racing thoughts. I winced every time her fingertips brushed across her piping hot coffee cup. Suddenly she reached out to pick up the cup, and instead she sent it flying with the back of her hand. Knocking things over is what we commonly call 'clumsiness'.

If you saw a blind man knock over a cup of coffee would you think of him as clumsy? No, because the 'awareness of surroundings' is obviously missing for him. The same would apply to a sighted person in a dark room. But I was sitting with my friend in broad daylight, and there

11

were no eyesight problems, illnesses, or injuries at play. Why then did she knock the cup flying?

The answer is that your body responds to what you're thinking about. Your nervous system contracts your muscles using the information from your thoughts. If you, the user, are thinking about being somewhere other than where you actually are, your body moves with conflicting information.

Have you ever knocked something over, stubbed your toe, or walked into the corner of a table? I know that I have many times, and it's always been when I wasn't paying attention to my actual surroundings. Everyone has the occasional uncoordinated movement, or moment of 'clumsiness'. When it's more than the occasional incident though, clumsiness can be a risky business. The following thoughts can lead to uncoordinated movements.

MULTI-TASKING: Thinking about doing more than one thing at the same time.

What we commonly refer to as 'multi-tasking' is a major cause of physical tension and suffering. When you think about performing an action, your nervous system is already responding to your thoughts. It doesn't differentiate between what you're actually doing, and something that you're only thinking about doing.

Research has confirmed that when a subject is only imagining himself to be running, his leg muscles begin to fire. Firing means that the signal is going to the muscle to cause it to contract. Therefore, if you're physically doing one thing, while also thinking about doing something else, your muscles will be firing erratically. Incidentally, you'll also be using more energy than you need to be at any given moment. Doing this for long periods of time can lead to chronic fatigue.

DAYDREAMING: Imagining yourself to be somewhere other than where you are.

Your body is responding to the circumstances around it based upon your thoughts. If you're thinking about being somewhere other than where you actually are, your body doesn't know the difference. For this reason you can be walking along daydreaming, and suddenly stumble into a hole in the ground that you didn't see coming.

When you're lounging on the couch daydreaming about a moonlight walk on the beach, your breathing slows down and your muscles relax. Try daydreaming instead about running down a dark alley with a monster on your heels. I don't think there'll be much relaxing going on! As the saying goes, 'be careful what you wish for'. Where your body is concerned your daydreams are wishes, and it will make every effort to fulfill them for you.

Daydreaming is a natural and mostly healthy process. There's no need to stop yourself from doing it, and you probably couldn't anyway. Do be aware though of what you're daydreaming about, and when; particularly if you think of yourself as being 'a little bit clumsy'. Make an effort to stay focused on what you're doing at the current moment. If you find this to be challenging, perhaps your problem is really something else entirely. It could be boredom, or a lack of passion in your life that is the culprit behind your clumsiness.

WORRYING: Thinking the worst about a situation in the future.

The act of worrying is imagining the worst possible outcome of a situation. It will usually be an outcome in which you see yourself losing something of value. This kind of destructive thinking puts you in fight-or-flight response, also known as stress. I refer to worrying as an action, because you're consciously choosing to pass your time doing it. You could just as easily choose to imagine the best possible outcome, and do that with your time instead.

If it gives you a feeling of security to prepare your home for a hurricane, or to lock your doors at night, then this isn't the same thing as worrying. To know the difference between 'being cautious' and 'worrying' ask yourself this question, 'Is thinking about this making me feel better, or worse?'

The stress of worrying can lead you to chronic and excessive muscle tension. It's difficult for your nervous system to coordinate movements correctly when you're continually in fight or flight response. If you're playing a game of cards, while at the same time thinking about getting fired from your job - watch out for that hot cup of coffee!

TEN WAYS TO IMPROVE COORDINATION

1. Next time you do something clumsy, notice what you were thinking and feeling directly before it happened.

2. Keep a note pad and pen with you at all times. Make notes about your coordination issues, and look for a pattern.

3. Stop multitasking! It may appear to you that you need to be multitasking to get through the day. This is an illusion of a cluttered mind. Even if you have three tasks on the go at once, you can still only do one thing at a time. If you decide to switch back and forth between projects, do so consciously. Focus only on what's in front of you; you'll get more done in the long run.

4. Use your daydreams to enhance the quality of your life. Keep your flights of fancy to times when you don't need your conscious mind fully engaged. Daydream away while you're creating a vision board, strolling on the beach, or soaking in the tub.

5. Take up pass-times or therapies that help you to unwind. Enjoy being fully in the moment with something like yoga, tai chi, or massage.

6. Realize that being clumsy is not who you are; it's something that you're doing. If you can determine the cause, you'll be able to do something about it.

7. If you already know, or suspect, that you're having trouble with your eyesight, then stop procrastinating. Get your vision checked out immediately.

8. When you catch yourself worrying about something - change your mind. Worrying has yet to prevent an upcoming disaster. Prepare for the future by all means, but always use your imagination to see the best possible outcome.

9. Slow down! You'll be surprised at how much more you'll achieve when you pace yourself. Taking your time can lead to fewer incidences of tripping, bumping, and knocking things over.

10. Stop labeling yourself. Every time you say, "I've always been clumsy" you're setting yourself up to have that experience again. Remember, as you think – so you move!

THE PAIN-CHAIN

Acute pain can stop you in your tracks, bring you to your knees, and even render you unconscious. When pain is acute there's no way that you'll be able to ignore it. Pain however, is far more than just a messenger telling you that your body's been injured. Burning, pinching, and aching can all be felt as a warning, long before an injury actually occurs.

The purpose of pain is to warn you that what you're doing is harmful, and that further damage is possible if you continue. When your mind and your body are working blissfully together, you'll be aware of the warning signals immediately. There'll be no delay between the first twinge of pain, and seeking the action that will bring relief.

When the initial warning twinges are ignored, your nervous system will attempt to correct the problem by sending backup signals. This will be felt as an urge to keep changing your position, or perhaps to avoid moving at all. Those seemingly insignificant twinges are the first link in your chronic pain chain. Every time you try to find relief, but are ignoring the original cause, you're creating another link. One pain leads to another, and your Chronic Pain Chain is forged!

Your automatic reaction to feeling pain is to tighten up. Your nervous system attempts to immobilize the joint, muscle, or ligament in danger of being damaged. If you ignore this reaction and keep on doing what you're doing, your own muscles will continue to fight you. As a result of this situation you'll experience impaired range-of-motion, weakness, and poor agility. Perhaps more importantly, you're at a greater risk for injury.

What do you do when you first wake up in the morning? Do you take in a deep breath and stretch your body as you breathe out? Or do you stumble out of bed and drag yourself to the kitchen for coffee? No matter what age you are at the moment, living with stiff sore and aching muscles may be normal for you, but it certainly isn't natural. Your body is an incredible machine, but it can only function using the information provided by you, the user.

Having been born with Palindromic Rheumatism, I began to forge my own chronic pain chains at an early age. My joints would take it in turns to swell up, and my muscles ached like a miserable toothache. The cold, wet days of my native England served only to aggravate this rare form of Rheumatoid Arthritis. There's no greater incentive to finding solutions to a problem, than to suffer with that problem yourself. For decades I've been observing what causes chronic pain, and discovering solutions that bring relief.

When a society becomes highly invested in technology, the individuals using it spend long periods of time sitting or standing still. Time itself becomes a precious commodity for commuters, and for people who are cramming their calendars full every day. The communication between the mind and the body is affected, and the result is millions of people living with chronic pain.

Your pain chain may have been forming insidiously for years. Chronic pain can be like a dripping tap that goes unnoticed until the water overflows. The cause of your pain may well be hiding in plain sight. The solution to the problem may also be right there in front of you, in what I call a 'realization blind spot'.

REALIZATION BLIND SPOTS

When you've illuminated all of your self-created blind spots, you'll experience a leap in personal evolution!

To call you a fool for creating your own chronic pain chain is to throw stones in a glass house. Everyone at some point has shifted around in an uncomfortable chair through an entire event. I'll even go out on a limb and say that we've all worn uncomfortable shoes, stayed out in the sun for too long, or slept in a poorly supported bed. Obviously there are reasons why you'd subject yourself to pain, even though they might not be immediately apparent. Here are just a few of them:

> Not wanting to hurt someone else's feelings
> Trying to avoiding embarrassment
> Laziness, indifference, or apathy
> Attempting to impress someone
> Feelings of guilt or obligation

Surely though, you'd always be aware of why you're choosing to put yourself in pain. If only it were that cut and dried. You've created a unique world for yourself out of your past experiences, current beliefs, and most daunting fears. Although what you're doing may appear to be a conscious act, there's more likely a less apparent subconscious motivation behind it. You may be being motivated by a thought behind the thought, so to speak.

I cleaned out my closet the other day, and took a practically new pair of shoes to the thrift shop. I remember what I told myself the day I bought those shoes, "So what if they pinch my toes, they look great! I'll just wear them when I don't have to walk very far." I wore them once. Today I no longer have that 'realization blind spot' when it comes to buying shoes. Take a look in your closet, and see what you can learn about yourself from what you find in there.

The solution to finding relief from your discomfort could be right in front of you, hidden by one of your own realization blind spots. You could be aware that you're hurting yourself on purpose, but not know why. It isn't necessary for you to delve into your subconscious to uncover your motivations. It may be enough to ask yourself these two questions:

> "What am I trying to achieve here, and who is it that I'm really trying to please?"

Wearing uncomfortable shoes is only one example of how you might be hurting yourself on purpose. This isn't just limited to women either. Realization blind spots can happen to anyone. They can make you miserable in your work life, at home, and even when you're working-out. Tennis courts, golf greens, running tracks, and gyms are all prime places for a realization blind spot to conceal self-inflicted pain.

If you're experiencing chronic pain in your life, then the chances are that you have at least one realization blind spot in effect. The first step to shedding light on those blind spots is to be aware that you have them. The second step is to realize that it doesn't always have to be this way. Things can change for the better!

CHANGING IT UP

A major realization blind spot that I frequently encounter is the belief that nothing is ever going to change. If you don't realize that your situation can improve, you'll not be making any effort to find solutions. If you want things in your life to change for the better, then you must first make changes in your life! One or more of the following beliefs could be blocking you from improving your condition:

I DON'T HAVE THE TIME OR THE MONEY TO CHANGE MY LIFE.

How much time and money do you currently spend on nonessential items in your life? How much time and money have you lost or wasted, because you were physically suffering in some way? Does your chronic pain cause you to miss work, or to lose out on time that you could be spending having fun?

This book is about helping you to uncover your blind spots; areas of your life where you may be causing your own problems. Finding the cause of your suffering need not cost you any more than you're spending right now. In fact finding *and removing* the cause of chronic pain, has the potential to save you a bundle on symptom relief.

You wouldn't be reading this book right now if you didn't still hope to find an answer somewhere. Realize right now that you already have all the time and money you need to make positive lifestyle changes. The rewards will be well worth it.

THERE CAN'T BE ANYTHING THAT I HAVEN'T ALREADY TRIED.

Have you already tried medication, surgery, physical therapy, chiropractic, acupuncture, yoga, Pilates, and everything else you can think of, yet still the pain persists?

What I'm sharing with you here isn't intended to be yet another form of treatment or management. The purpose of this book is to uncover the causes of your chronic pain-chain, and to create solutions that will remove the problem at its source. It's basically a three step process:

ONE: Pinpoint the origin of the problem
TWO: Find and implement a solution
THREE: Break the chronic pain-chain

I'LL ONLY TRY IT IF MY INSURANCE COVERS IT.

There are many forms of natural healing services available that aren't even recognized by insurance companies. I alone have three decades of experience uncovering the causes of chronic pain. I've spent that time creating and implementing my own solutions for relief. The combinations of techniques that I've developed over the years don't fall under any state or federal regulations. Therefore, the work that I do with clients isn't covered by insurance.

If you discover a therapy that you think might help you, ask for testimonials. Read what other people have to say about their experience with that service. Don't be afraid to ask the therapist questions. Learn as much as you can about applying that service to your particular needs. Your insurance company may cover many types of therapy, but that's no guarantee that one of them is the right one for you.

Your body wants to be at ease. It seeks to be in its natural state of wellbeing. Your nervous system will continue to send you, the user, feedback to help you get to that place. Let me ask you a question. Would you drive around with your car engine clunking and misfiring? I'd go out on a limb and say that you wouldn't. You'd take it to several mechanics if necessary, until somebody figured out what was causing the problem.

Without uncovering the cause of a problem, there can really be no lasting relief. Have faith; be determined; do whatever it takes for you to shed light on your realization blind spots. Through finding and implementing your own personal solutions, you can positively make changes in your life. The guide to finding those solutions may not be in your insurance company's reference book.

ILLNESS, INJURY, AND 'OTHER'

Medical professionals do a fabulous job, but they're trained to treat medical conditions. Not all chronic pain is caused by an illness or injury that requires medical treatment. Millions of people every year are suffering with chronic pain being caused by realization blind spots. Blind spots don't need to be treated, they just need to be realized and addressed.

For example, Jane Doe breaks her right leg and her doctor puts it in a cast for six weeks. Once the cast comes off, Jane undergoes six weeks of physical therapy for the injured leg. The leg is rehabilitated, and she resumes her daily life. The parts of Jane's body however, work together to mobilize her; no one part works by itself.

Jane has now developed painful tension in her right shoulder from leaning on the crutch. Also, her left hip is aching after having to support her weight since the accident. Jane now has two chronic tension problems that left unheeded will continue to grow. No matter how fit she becomes in the future, Jane will be dragging those pain chains around until she addresses the underlying imbalances.

Another consideration is that an accident usually doesn't 'just happen'. Specific circumstances can lead up to a trip and fall. Perhaps Jane already had tight or weak muscles that were causing her balance issues. The problem may have been poor eyesight affecting her perception of depth. The period following an injury is an excellent time to reevaluate your lifestyle, and your current physical condition.

Your body has an incredible ability to heal itself, with or without your conscious help. If the cause of your pain chain is still there though, you'll continue to suffer the consequences. Addressing only the symptoms won't break the chain. Recovering from an injury may well just create another link. The way to uncover the underlying problem is through observation, knowledge, and understanding of how your particular body works.

Emotional pain can lead to physical pain, and vice versa. Your body is the hardware, your nervous system is the software, and your mind is the user. If 'the user' programs the software with flawed or incorrect information, then the hardware can't be expected to work properly. The reverse of this is also true. If your body is injured or out of balance, the feelings of pain and restriction will impact the comfort level of your everyday life. Try as you might, you just can't ignore your own body language.

BODY LANGUAGE

Once a blind spot has been uncovered, it doesn't need to be treated per se. Chronic pain can result from being ignorant of the common causes of the 'pain chain'. Once you've identified the underlying cause, all you have to do is remove it. For example, if your back pain is being caused by a chair with poor lumbar support, then get a better chair. The chain must be broken at the cause before stretching and strengthening exercises can restore balance.

The cause of your pain may not be as simple as a poorly supporting chair though. Your belief systems and your view of the world are constantly being expressed in how you sit and stand. Every move that you make tells a story about your lifestyle. How you hold your posture speaks volumes about the level of your confidence. When you enter a room, your expectations are displayed in the way that you walk.

In 1979 I attended a workshop for hypnotherapists in Northampton, England. The title of the workshop was 'Body Language'. The program was designed to teach the attendees how to 'read between the lines' in a client consultation. They taught us to recognize when a person is telling us something that's in conflict with his or her body language. They also imparted that body language reflects a deeper thought process, and is therefore a more genuine communication.

24

Your emotions are the result of what you choose to think and believe. Certain thoughts such as anxiety and anger have an obvious effect on the body. It can be a little bit different for each person, but feelings of anger typically lead to a flushed face, a raised voice, or a clenched jaw. These kinds of physical manifestations are hard to miss. For me personally, when I'm feeling anxious about something like taking an exam, I get an upset stomach. Even if I'm not the one being tested, I can easily be anxious on behalf of someone else!

Anxiety and anger are emotional responses being stimulated in the present moment. They may well be related to subconscious fears or interpretations, but the response is stimulated by a situation happing in the moment. This makes it easier to identify such emotions. Not all thought patters are that overtly expressed though. Some habits of thought and their emotional responses are much more difficult to recognize.

Believing that you're being victimized by a relative, a company, the government, or anyone else, is rarely going to be a single situation response. Such thinking and its related feelings are typically internalized, and can lead to some heavy chronic pain chains. Someone chronically thinking of his or her self as a victim will sit, or stand with arms crossed over the ribs, and chest slummed forward. Adopting this position can lead to impaired breathing, low energy, and backache.

No matter what your thoughts and corresponding emotions may be, your body is always re-acting to that information. Your thoughts don't have to be unconscious and habitually negative. You have the ability to think whatever you choose. It's not necessary to re-write the thought patterns in your subconscious. Just use your mind and body connection to create new ones. Cultivate positive subconscious thoughts by choosing to animate your body as if you already have.

Think for a moment about how a person would sit and stand if he or she were calm, relaxed, and confident. That person will have a straight back; ribcage lifted allowing the diaphragm to expand for a full breath. His shoulders will be gently back and relaxed, expressing confidence without aggression. Her facial muscles will be softened with a slight smile, and her hands will be resting in her lap. If you're not already communicating with calm, relaxed, and confident body language, start right now.

I think it's great if you're all excited about life-style changes that include exercise, and a healthier diet. But before you embark on that journey you need to get what I'm saying here about body language. Every thought you have leads to muscle contractions, hormone production, and the next thought that's going to impact your body. The mind and body connection isn't just new-age fluff; it's a scientific fact, and the foundation for chronic pain relief.

Take a step back for a moment, and look at the relationships in your life. Ask yourself if you're expecting someone else to change his or her behavior to suit you. Consider the logic of refusing to accept a policy that's already in place, just because you don't agree with it. If there's one thing that you can always control in your life – it's whether or not you choose to struggle.

Let me define here what I mean by 'struggle'. You're struggling when you resent what's already happened in the past. You're struggling when you complain about what's currently happening in the present. You're struggling when you worry about what's about to happen in the future. If you want to enjoy more fun in your life, then you'll need to go with the flow.

Imagine what it would feel like to always expect the most positive results. Imagine yourself always standing tall, calm, and relaxed. Doing so may not change your outward circumstances, but it will positively change your inward experience. When you decide to act out of conscious decision in every circumstance, it can be blissfully liberating. If you want to feel at ease in your body, you'll first need to take responsibility for your thoughts.

YOUR FURNITURE – FRIEND OR FOE?

What percentage of your day do you spend sitting down? Include sitting on a couch, dining chair, armchair, recliner, patio seat, office chair, car seat, and or in a bus. Studies have concluded that an average person spends between fifty to seventy percent of the day sitting. In my experience of working with clients, that percentage is often higher!

Seventy percent of your day is quite a chunk of time to spend suspended by your buttocks, with your legs dangling from your pelvis. The human body just isn't designed to sit in chairs. If you were to visit countries in the East, you'd find people either standing or sitting crossed legged on the ground, even while they're eating.

In recent times the west has gained more influence in these eastern countries. Sitting on chairs has become more common now, and along with it so has chronic pain. The problem with sitting can be exacerbated by generic furniture. No matter how expensive or well-made your furnishings may be, there can be no one piece that fits all body sizes.

Furniture that's not fully and correctly supporting you is harming you. In my experience few people take the time to find that perfect fit. On the contrary, the majority are oblivious to the important role that furniture plays in his or her life. When I raise the subject, there are two excuses that I commonly hear for hanging on to ill-fitting, or worn out seating. The first excuse is that he or she doesn't have the time to shop for furniture. The second is that there isn't any money in the budget for it.

If you're using one or both of these excuses, then I invite you to examine your priorities. In the past few weeks have you done anything on the following list?

Went to the movies
Got your nails done
Watched a live sport
Had dinner at a restaurant

    Traded in a perfectly good car
    Bought a pair of non-essential shoes
    Had electrolysis, or wax hair removal
    Bought a piece of non-essential clothing
    Bought a new TV, Blueray, or Sound System
    Bought an animal from a breeder instead of rescuing one
    Put money into a savings account to be used for a rainy day

Ill fitting, worn out, or broken furniture is far worse than a rainy day. Ignoring it is akin to ignoring an insidious leak under your kitchen floor. Sooner or later something is going to give way, and the cost will be immense!

There's an old saying in England, "save a penny, and spend a pound." It means that when you try to save money by not fixing something, you end up spending far more in the long run. This is true with the furniture that supports your precious body. If you continue to sleep in a bed that's shaped like a ladle, you'll end up sinking your money into chronic pain management.

It isn't necessary to understand anatomy to find the right support for your body. Your head needs to sit squarely on your shoulders for your neck muscles to be in balance. Therefore, if you're sitting or lying for long periods of time with your chin tilted up, or down, you're creating incorrect tension in your neck muscles. This can lead to periodic or continuous dull aching, or sharp shooting pains in your neck and shoulders.

If you're not sitting upright, then you need to have your head supported. This will allow your neck muscles to relax. Buy a new arm chair, or a couch with a high back that supports your head in line with your body. Raise or lower your TV if it isn't already at eye level. Use cushions or pillows behind your head and shoulders, so that you can relax when you sit back. It may be an inconvenience to shop for cushions, or to rearrange your furniture. But how convenient is it to live with chronic pain?

Everyone has a unique body shape. Nonetheless, every spine is basically the same. Your backbone is gently curved to buffer the shock and stress of movement. The lumbar area is your lower back at the top of your buttocks. This part of your spine is the most flexible, and carries the majority of your body weight. For this reason the lumbar spine is prone to strains, sprains, and disc injuries. Sitting poorly supported even for a short period of time, can only add to this burden.

To protect your lumber spine you'll need to be either sitting upright, or to be resting back onto a chair without slumping. Looking directly forward while sitting in a slouched position causes you to lift your chin, and shorten the back of your neck. This particular posture is common with anyone who works at a computer. It's also a major cause of chronic pain in the neck, back, and shoulders.

Trunk muscles that are strained and out of balance due to poor posture, become chronically tight and weak. The result is a lack of the strength and flexibility needed to support your lower back. The muscles of your trunk are involved in everyday movements such as twisting, bending, and lifting something up. Imbalance in your trunk muscles therefore, can not only lead to chronic pain but can also lead to an injury.

To be completely relaxed while sitting at your computer you'll need your chin to be at a right angle to your neck. Your eyes will be looking straight ahead. If you're looking down at your screen, either lower your chair, or put your monitor on a stand. If you don't have a monitor stand then be creative; use a telephone book instead. If you're looking up at your screen, either raise your chair, or sit on a cushion.

Both the heels and toes of your feet need to be fully supported and preferably resting on the ground. Position your thighs to be parallel with the floor beneath you. This will prevent the weight of your legs from pulling down on your lower back. If your seat is too high and for some reason you can't lower it, use a footstool or books to achieve the required support.

If you're concerned about the cost of a professional ergonomical assessment, do your own assessment based on the information given above. It may not be necessary at all for you to buy a new chair or special equipment to fix your furniture woes. Something as simple as a small cushion, or a rolled towel could be all the additional lumber support that you need.

My friend Tammy had been suffering with tears of pain at the end of her work day for years. The company that she worked for had invested in buying her a new and expensive office chair. Unfortunately, this is usually the first and only attempt to fix such a problem. Often, as in Tammy's case, this doesn't help at all. The reason is that the lumbar support is still in the wrong place.

Tammy had been afraid to make any more noise about her chronic back pain. Her concern was that any further ergonomic equipment would have to be paid for out of her own pocket. I did for Tammy what I always do; I looked around for something with which to rig the chair. In the kitchen I came across a plastic tablecloth; it was perfect. Five minutes later the cloth was rolled up and attached to Tammy's brand new office chair with a large rubber band. Her pain relief was instantaneous!

Expensive furniture is not synonymous with comfort. An ergonomic assessment is not necessarily going to break the bank. Knowledge, awareness, and action are worth far more to you than a posh director's chair when it comes to pain relief. The correct fit is what's necessary to break the pain chains caused by your furniture foes.

WORN DOWN SHOES

Wearing worn down shoes causes a vicious cycle situation. When your hip muscles are tight or weak, you walk with an incorrect movement pattern. This in turn affects your ankles, and begins to wear down the sides of your shoes.

30

Wearing worn down shoes reinforces this incorrect movement pattern. Do you see the problem here?

Check your shoes on a regular basis for uneven wearing of the soles. You may find that you consistently wear down either the inside, or the outside of every pair of your shoes. If you find this happening to you, then take action to remedy the situation. Your expensive shoes can be taken to the cobblers to be built up again. Inexpensive shoes are best to be replaced altogether.

Chronic knee pain can result from walking on the outside, or the inside of your feet. The problem could be due to weak ankles. When your ankles collapse inwards it causes you to invert your feet. This ankle weakness is often mistaken for just being 'flat footed'. When your weak ankle muscles lead to an outward collapse, you'll tend to walk on the outer edges of your feet. Fixing or getting rid of problem shoes will be a major step to strengthening your ankle muscles correctly.

Wearing shoes that have worn down unevenly is counterproductive to any stretching that you're doing for your hips. You'll be attempting to create balanced muscle tension, while still reinforcing an imbalance every time you walk. By checking that your shoes are wearing down evenly, you'll be helping to relieve chronic pain in both your hips and your knees.

THE NATURE OF HEALING HABITS

Habits aren't intrinsically a bad thing to have. It's the habits that are causing you harm that are bad. Once you realize that you can consciously create habitual behavior that supports your wellness, the word itself takes on a whole new meaning. This realization can be found in understanding the difference between a habit, and a natural instinctive response.

A habit is something that you originally chose to do one time. Then you decided to do it again, and again, until it became a semi-conscious behavior. For example, I owned my first car before the invention of keyless locking mechanisms. I developed a habit of flipping the lock on the driver's side door as I was getting out of the vehicle.

The car I have today has a handheld remote. Yet still I'm locking the door on the inside by hand as I'm climbing out. Unfortunately, locking the driver's side door in my present ride locks all of the doors simultaneously. This particular habit could cost me a bill from a locksmith, should I accidentally leave my keys inside the car!

Conversely, a natural instinct is an unconscious protective response. When dirt flies up into your face you instinctively blink to protect your eyes. This reaction isn't a form of habit, but if it was it would be a good one to have! To improve your body's ability to heal itself, nurture habits that mimic or improve upon your natural instincts.

When you feel a twinge of pain, or a nagging ache, do you automatically reach for an over-the-counter pill? If the answer to this question is 'yes', then you may have a blind spot when it comes to trying other options first. Non-prescription medications may be readily available, but that doesn't make them free of harmful side effects.

TURNING A NATURAL INSTINCT INTO A GOOD HABIT

Palindromic Rheumatism causes one or more joints to arbitrarily swell for days at a time. The pressure on the joint causes chronic pain, and the muscles around the area ache continuously. Having been born with this condition, I decided years ago not to rely on pain medications for relief. As I'm allergic to anti-inflammatory medications, my drug options have been somewhat limited anyway.

The field of Homeopathy offers alternatives to some pharmaceuticals. It was a massage therapist who first introduced me to Triflora, a homeopathic remedy for arthritis and tendinitis. Applying this topical cream brings me blessed relief from the misery of rheumatism. Gently rubbing Triflora into my aching muscles also has an additional benefit: the healing power of touch.

Think for a moment; what's the first thing you do when you get a sudden twinge of pain? Your instinct is to put your hand over the area that's hurting. The reason could be that the sensation of touch sends pleasant, non-painful signals to the nervous system; your palm and fingers feel warm and soothing. Additionally, your hand is immobilizing and protecting the area from further harm.

You can take the instinct to put your hand on a place that hurts, and turn it into a good habit. Creating new good habits is more productive, and ultimately more successful, than trying to break bad habits. Next time your chronic pain chain begins to rattle, try doing the following before resorting to something else:

ONE: Place your hand on the painful joint or muscle, and keep it there.
TWO: Sit down, and be consciously calm and still.
THREE: Take in a deep breath, and relax as you breathe out (more about breathing later).
FOUR: Focus your attention on soothing and relaxing the painful area.

FIVE: Feel the warm sensation of your palm, and imagine the pain just melting away.

You can choose to create a good habit out of doing the above. If the pain doesn't then begin to subside, you can choose what you want to do next. Before automatically reaching for an outside remedy, give your body a chance to respond naturally. I've been using the healing benefits of touch for years, expecting the pain to diminish. And for me it usually does.

I taught this simple technique to my mother after she banged her arthritic knuckles on the door jamb. A couple of minutes later she exclaimed that the pain was going away. "When I've knocked my knuckles like that before," she told me, "it's hurt me for hours!"

Although it may not be a cure for arthritis or rheumatism, using your instinct to touch where it hurts can break your chronic pain-chain. Focusing on pain can cause it to feel even worse. What you put your attention on becomes the center of your experience. Place your attention instead on your breathing, and on the warmth of your hand. Sometimes it's the simplest techniques that can afford the most thankful relief.

The response to a back twinge is another instinct that forms a good habit. Sitting or standing with poor posture is a precursor to a sudden twinge of pain. When a back muscle spasms your instinctive response is to straighten up. This happens automatically to allow your back to relax. Tight back muscles can also cause a dull continuous ache. The response is the same; you feel the need to sit up straight.

To resist your natural instinct is a bad habit to form. So is going right back to what caused the problem in the first place. Find yourself a chair to sit in that supports your head, shoulders, and lumbar area correctly. Take a few deep breaths, and allow your body to release the death grip on your muscles. No matter what you were doing before now, responding positively to your pain signals will be well worth the effort.

When the tension just won't release, lie down on your back on the floor or bed. Rest your arms beside your body, and legs uncrossed. Place cushions or rolled up towels under your head and knees if needed for added comfort. In yoga this is called Savasana (Corpse Pose), and it's considered the most important pose to practice. You don't need flexibility, strength, or balance in this position. You can quiet your mind, and relax every muscle in your body. Lie still for at least five minutes, taking slow deep and relaxing breaths.

If you're at work and have to stay in your chair, you can still follow your natural instinct to sit up straight and relax. Sit back in your chair for a few minutes, and allow your muscles to release the excess tension. Lift your ribcage, and give your lower back a chance to let go. Take a few deep breaths; breathe both in and out through your nose. While you're relaxing, think about how you can make improvements to your chair or work-station. Be proactive in preventing another link from being added to your pain chain.

TAMING THE TENSION

Tension in itself isn't a problem. If you didn't maintain a certain level of muscle tension, you'd flop on the ground like a noodle. The problem arises when certain muscles become chronically tight or weak, or are contracting out of sequence. Whether you're sitting standing or bending over, to maintain good posture your muscle tension needs to be in balance.

There are three main causes of incorrect muscle tension. Each one can be a part of your everyday activities. When you're doing something every day, the incorrect tension pattern builds up slowly and insidiously. By the time a pain chain becomes apparent, the daily activity behind it doesn't appear to be related to it at all.

FIGHT OR FLIGHT RESPONSE

The first cause of incorrect muscle tension is being in a fight-or-flight response all day. When faced with a sudden fright or an imminent danger, the natural response is to either run or fight. In nature you only have a few minutes, if that, to get away or to win the battle to survive. Whether you like it or not you're an animal, just like that deer in the headlights. Your nervous system responds to your thoughts of danger by increasing your heart rate, switching you to mouth breathing, and causing your muscles to increase the tension.

Wild animals such as deer have an advantage over humans; they live their lives entirely in the present moment. Non-human animals only respond to danger when the threat is actually imminent. Humans on the other hand dwell on the past, and imagine all kinds of dangers for the future to come. Fight-or-flight is a safety response to a present danger, and is supposed to pass quickly. When you allow fearful thoughts to bombard your nervous system all day long, you create a situation known as 'stress'.

The blind spot here is the belief that your thoughts are automatic responses to situations. In reality, situations are subjective; they only exist because you think about them. Stress can be relieved simply by realizing that you can change your mind at any time. The following thoughts keep you in fight-or-flight response, and can lead to chronic stress:

> *I'm never going to finish on time.*
> *I'll get fired if I can't do this.*
> *I'm never going to get a raise.*
> *How can I get everything done in one day?*
> *I hate my boss.*

The following are thoughts that create ease, and can release chronic stress:

> *I'll do the best that I can in the time that I have left.*
> *If I get fired because I can't do this, I'm in the wrong job anyway.*
> *I can either choose to appreciate what I earn, or I can look for another job.*
> *I'll get a lot more done if I focus on just one thing at a time.*
> *I don't agree with my boss, but my life will be easier if I accept his authority.*

Stress can easily become chronic when it's connected to the fear of losing something. Fear such as this is subconscious, and can be difficult to recognize. It may sound cliché to say that it dates back to your childhood, but it usually does. If you're feeling that your life is chronically stressful, then see if you can figure out what it is that you're afraid of losing.

How would you feel if you lost your job; are you afraid of having no livelihood? Is it important to you that the people you work with show you respect? Are you afraid of losing someone in your life who shows you love, praise, acceptance, or something else of value? Continuing to struggle with such fears can only lead to more suffering. This kind of danger only exists in your imagination. Being clear about this is a big step towards letting go of the tension in your life.

STILL LIFE

Before the age of technology was created, jobs in general were more physically demanding. Farmers toiled in fields. Secretaries walked to the file rooms. Day to day life was all about movement. Today it's quite possible to live your entire life – work, home, and social – from the comfort of your cell phone.

Professions have become so specialized, and departmentalized, that we're becoming little more than piece-workers. Each person fulfilling a small role in the production that makes up his or her own industry. Whether you consider this to be an evolutionary step up or not is irrelevant. How it's particularly affecting your body, well this is absolutely relevant to your personal level of fitness.

As technology makes everything accessible in one place, the need to interact with other people is minimized. The work environment is becoming more like still-life. The sitting, standing, and bending in one position that is so often required today, leads to muscles that are chronically short and tight. This chronic tension in turn leads to discomfort and poor agility.

Professionals such as surgeons, dentists, and gardeners spend long periods of time bent over. Hairdressers, painters, and electricians hold their arms out for longer than is ideally comfortable. Positioning the body in this way causes tension pain in the neck and shoulders. This is because the muscles of the neck and shoulders are working overtime to extend the arms against gravity. Last but not least are the drivers, jockeys, and desk bound workers all creating their own individual tension issues.

The situation can be exacerbated if your hobbies are a continuation of still-life activities. Do you relax when you get home with a good book or a movie? Is knitting or sewing something that you enjoy after work hours? Take a moment to consider how much activity your body actually gets to enjoy each day. If nothing else, at least go for a walk before you sit down to spend more time being still.

REPEATING YOURSELF

The third major cause of incorrect and chronic muscle tension is repetitive motion. The pain caused by doing something the same way, over and over again, can be felt as dull, aching, sharp, or burning. The type of discomfort experienced will depend on the movement, and the muscles involved. Anyone who spends their time typing, golfing, bowling, playing tennis or soccer, sewing, knitting, or writing, knows all too well the consequences of repetitive motion.

There are many other causes however, of repetitive motion pain that aren't so quickly or commonly recognized. Reaching for a telephone over and over again in the same place at work can lead to chronic shoulder pain. Turning the wheel on a sewing machine, or a microscope can eventually lead not only to pain, but to functional problems with the wrist or thumb.

My client's chronic back pain was being caused by picking up her grandson's toys off the floor every day; not to mention picking up the toddler himself. Walking around with a baby sitting on one hip is a recipe for long term discomfort. The pain caused by weeding in the garden for hours can also be linked to repetitive motion. The pain is exacerbated if the motion is also one of squatting or bending incorrectly.

The repetitive actions need not necessarily be performed one directly after the other. If the action itself is out of balance and causing strain, just doing it once a day will be enough to lead to chronic pain. For example: sitting in the front seat of the car and reaching around for a bag that's in the back seat. Climbing out of the car itself can also lead to problems if you shift all of your weight onto one leg. The pain may not necessarily be felt in the hip; it may be experienced as lower back pain. Turn your body when you get out of the car, and use both legs to support yourself.

Your brain stores movement patterns to make life easier for you. When the patterns are causing strain, your muscles and tendons will send signals to you – the user - that they're under stress. This communication will be experienced as pain or discomfort. Pain is a warning that something is wrong, and if you're paying attention it will be felt *before* an injury occurs.

Have you been ignoring that occasional twinge, or persistent ache? Have you been losing your balance, favoring one leg, or feeling stiff after sitting for a while? These are warning signs to let you know that problem patterns have already formed. If you ignore these warnings and do nothing about them, the problems will only continue to get worse.

Pay attention to what you do repetitively in your everyday life, and make the necessary changes to ease the tension. Move the telephone closer to you. Reorganize your desk or end table if that's what it takes. Sit on a stool to weed your garden, or pay a few dollars to a high school student to help you. These changes could be so simple to implement, yet the relief that you feel could well be tremendous!

TWELVE COMMON CAUSES OF PAINFUL TENSION

This list is compiled from working with clients that were found to be causing their own chronic pain problem. Nothing on the following list is a medical condition, or related to an injury of any kind. These people had been suffering with chronic pain for years, having no idea that the root cause was just a realization blind spot!

1. Playing golf, tennis, or bowling without stretching correctly afterwards
2. Carrying a purse, computer, or any other kind of bag on one shoulder
3. Reaching to the back seat of the car to pull a bag onto the front seat

4. Driving with one hand on the wheel, and the arm straight and tense

5. Having a TV or a monitor positioned above, or below eye level

6. Sitting on a chair so high that the heels don't touch the ground

7. Sitting with one foot resting on the knee of the opposite leg

8. Standing with more weight on one foot than on the other

9. Holding the telephone between the ear and the shoulder

10. Sleeping with the head resting on an upstretched arm

11. Exercising one muscle group and ignoring another

12. Driving with the elbow resting on the window sill

If you believe that you've developed something like tennis elbow or carpal tunnel syndrome, then a visit to the doctor may be in order. Acute tendonitis could need medical attention. If in doubt, get it checked out by a physician just to be sure. Whether you've already developed tendinitis or not though, taking action to address the cause of chronic pain is still a wise choice. Eliminating or correcting the twelve actions on the previous list could simply help to relieve the suffering in your life.

PLANTAR FASCIITIS

The plantar fascia is a strip of connective tissues that runs along the bottom of your foot. Plantar fasciitis can be very painful, and can make it difficult for you to put your weight down on your heels. Unless you spend your life with your feet propped up this will affect how you walk, and can only lead to further problems. One of the most common causes of Plantar Fasciitis is wearing flip-flops. Any type of strapless sandal will cause you to contract the bottoms of your feet as you're walking in them.

Your physician can diagnose the symptoms, and there are treatments such as cortisone shots and physical therapy. If allowed to progress unchecked however, plantar fasciitis can lead to heel spurs – a very painful condition that could require surgery. Quite often though, the beginning pain signals of plantar fasciitis are aggravating, but not enough to warrant a doctor's visit. In a circumstance such as this, I use what I call my 'pain scale'.

The 'pain scale' runs from one to ten. Determine where on the pain scale your current pain level is falling. Let's say for example that the pain in the bottom of your right foot is currently a five. Next you decide which action you're going to take to relieve the pain. You could choose to massage the bottoms of your feet with massage oil, three times a day for five days. If at the end of the fifth day the pain has dropped to a four, then the action is effective. You'll continue with the massage until the pain drops to a zero.

For this particular type of chronic pain, gentle stretching of the bottoms of the feet and toes can also help to relieve the plantar fascia. Not to forget that tight calf muscles can affect the feet as well. The gastrocnemius, commonly referred to as the 'gastroc', is the muscle that looks like a pair of avocados between the back of your knee and your ankle. These muscles play a small role in plantar flexion (pointing your toes away from you).

People with short gastroc muscles will find it difficult to build bulk in the calves. I'm one of these people myself. I can do calf raises until I'm blue in the face, and I'll still look like a lanky stork! Conversely, people with long gastroc muscles can bulk up easily; even if they don't work out much at all. Therefore, the way that your calf muscles look is not necessarily an indication as to how strong or tight they may be. A little gentle stretching often is worth more, and is much safer, than aggressive stretching once in a while. The gastroc is more effectively stretched when your leg is straight.

The calf muscles that are more directly associated with pointing your toes away from you are the soleus muscles. A tight soleus muscle can add to irritation of the heel, and cause tension under the foot. The soleus muscles are stretched with the knee in a bent position. A simple way to see if you have tight soleus muscles is to lie on your stomach, with your knees bent to ninety degrees. If you can easily pull your toes down towards your knees and feel a stretch in the calf, then you're good to go. If not, then gentle stretching of the soleus may be in order for you.

If you have a realization blind spot about pain in your heels, or the bottoms of your feet, now is the time to do something about it. Chronic pain caused by incorrect movement patterns doesn't just go away by itself. Gentle stretching and self-massage can be excellent steps to take towards finding relief. Perhaps even more important, keep your flip-flops aside for wearing at the beach. Investing in sandals with supporting ankle straps will help to break the pain chain.

NECK TENSION HEADACHES

Have you ever watched a butterfly flittering around a bush? It doesn't just fly up and down, or left and right; its aeronautic agility is amazing. To accurately follow the unpredictable path of a butterfly, you'll need to move your head around in its full range-of-motion. Fortunately, the agility of your neck is equally amazing.

Many jobs today require the head to remain in a fixed position for long periods of time. Eyes looking directly forward, glued to the TV or computer screen. Sitting slumped over adds to the tension of keeping your head in one place for long periods. A hunched back and rounded shoulders causes you to lift your chin up to look straight ahead. Tilting your head back in this position shortens the muscles in the back of your neck, and weakens the muscles in the front. This imbalance of muscle tension is a major cause of headaches.

Look at the picture of a skeleton in an anatomy book; the back and neck are upright, and the head is sitting squarely on top of the shoulders. Ideally, your skeleton would look like this too. To balance the muscle tension in your neck, first correct your posture using the information previously given. Check the position of your computer screen and your office chair, and correct them if necessary. It may be difficult at first to sit up straight. Using the muscles in your back this way could feel as if you've been working out!

A warm compress on the back of your neck and shoulders may help to relieve muscle tension. You can buy a hot pack that can be warmed in the microwave at most local pharmacies. Sit with your head and shoulders well supported, and take a few deep breaths while you relax. Avoid using a cold pack unless you've been directed to do so by your physician. Cold is used to reduce the swelling when there's an injury. If the pain or discomfort is due to tight muscles only, and there's definitely no injury, then heat is more likely to be effective.

Sitting up correctly day-to-day may be all that's needed to balance the tension in your neck muscles. You won't find out though unless you make the effort. A simple exercise that you can perform for your neck is called 'following the butterfly'. Please note that if you feel any pinching, burning, tingling, or any other unexpected sensation when moving your head, consult your physician before trying this, or any other form of exercise.

Sit up straight and close your eyes. Imagine that you're watching a butterfly moving in slow motion. Watch the beautiful colored wings flittering around you in all directions. Follow its ever changing movements slowly with your chin - not with your eyes. Slightly part your teeth and relax your jaw. Carefully move your head in its full natural range-of-motion, no straining. Take deep slow breaths, and relax your shoulders throughout the exercise.

As you follow the butterfly in your mind, imagine yourself being outside on a lovely day. How good it feels to be chilling out and relaxing for a change. There's an old saying that's been around for generations, "stop and smell the roses". More recently the saying has mutated into, "stop and smell the coffee". It's a sad sign of our times that even a break is now taken indoors, and often spent reading, or 'surfing the web'. If you suffer from neck tension headaches, look around you. You may be amazed at what you've been missing!

EYE TENSION HEADACHES

Arguably the most neglected muscles in the body are those of the eyes. Even though eyestrain is commonly recognized as a cause of headaches, the solution that usually springs to mind is a new pair of glasses. Of course it makes sense to get your eyes tested, particularly if you haven't done so for years. It also makes sense to relax the extraocular muscles of your overworked eyes.

The average day calls for you to look at something close-up and stationary for hours at a time. This causes your eye muscles to shorten, creating excessive tension. Imagine sitting with your elbow bent all day. How do you think it would feel when you finally stretched your arm out again?

You don't need a lot of time or special equipment to exercise your eyes. You don't even need to get out of your seat. A simple routine will stretch the muscles that control your windows to the world. Whether you're getting headaches or not, it'll benefit you to focus on eye exercises – if you'll excuse the pun. The following is a sequence that I learned in yoga training to relieve the muscle tension of the eyes:

ONE: Sit comfortably and well supported with your shoulders relaxed.
TWO: Cup the palms of your hands over your eyes.
THREE: Close the edges so that no light is visible with your eyes open.
FOUR: Look into the darkness, and imagine that you're looking at a mountain far away.
FIVE: Imagine the fields and forests between you and the mountain. See the blue sky and the puffy clouds above the peaks, far off on the horizon.

SIX: Stare at the image in your imagination for at least thirty seconds. If you find it difficult to imagine the scene, just think about the last time you looked at something far away.

SEVEN: Next, close your eyes and slowly take your hands away.

EIGHT: Now blink your eyes rapidly for about three seconds.

NINE: Squeeze your eyes closed again and hold for three more seconds, then release.

TEN: Finally, take in a deep breath, and as you breathe out relax your eyes completely.

If you're fortunate enough to have a beautiful view outside your window, take the time to gaze outside and expand your vision. If not, just look around you at all there is to see in the room. Then keeping your head still, slowly look to your left, then right, and then up, and then down. Be careful not to move your head, only your eyes. Next, see how much detail you can pick up using just your peripheral vision.

If you suffer from eye tension headaches, imagine living in a world of darkness. Learn to appreciate everything that you see, and take the time to look long and linger. Your own mind is your most powerful pain reliever.

MIND HOW YOU STRETCH

In the world of personal training and athletic coaching, there's a great deal of controversy about the benefits of stretching. Lengthening chronically short muscles, increasing blood flow, and relaxing painful tension are all recognized benefits. The controversy lies around whether stretching can be detrimental in sporting activities, rather than enhancing performance.

Many professional organizations, including the American College of Sports Medicine, have done studies on the detriments versus benefits of stretching. The results have often been contradictory. I noticed when reading these studies that they're all about the physical results of when, and how long to stretch muscles. It's clear to me why the results are contradictory. The studies are being done on the act of stretching, not on the principle of flexibility.

Now-a-days the word 'stretching' inspires in people visions of lean bodies contorting themselves on yoga sticky mats. Ironically, the reason I hear most often for avoiding yoga practice is that he or she doesn't have enough flexibility. The science of yoga approaches flexibility through understanding that it's a practice of the mind, not just a function of the body. When your mind and body are in perfect sync, you'll naturally recognize the impulse to stretch when it's necessary.

It used to be as natural for humans as it is for cats to stretch-out upon waking from a deep sleep. That stretch reflex has been mostly buried today under piles of mental clutter. A daily stretching routine can go a long way to easing your muscle tension problems. Stretching incorrectly however, can aggravate an issue that's already causing you to suffer. Ironically, incorrect stretching could actually be adding hefty links to your chronic pain-chain, rather than breaking it.

BREATHING

Learning how to breathe correctly is the first step to reawakening your natural stretch reflex. Breathing is a communicator between your mind and your body. Becoming consciously aware of your breath is paramount to chronic pain relief, and also to flexibility. Begin by paying attention to whether you're breathing through your nose or your mouth. It's natural to breathe through your nose, both in and out, when you're feeling safe and relaxed. Breathing through your nose does the following for you:

1. Warms the air to the correct temperature for your lungs
2. Filters out dust particles, allergens, and other impurities
3. Signals your nervous system that 'all is well' in your world

If allergies are preventing you from breathing through your nose, I suggest that you pay a visit to your physician. It will benefit you to resolve any issue that causes you to breathe through your mouth. Mouth breathing and holding your breath are both part of the fight-or-flight response - they're both signs of stress. Your mind and your body are constantly communicating with each other. Therefore, no matter what the cause may be, if your breathing mimics the stress response your nervous system will be responding accordingly.

Although respiration is autonomic, your breathing rhythms are also responding to what you're thinking. If you're feeling tense and you want to relax, then consciously breathe as you would if you were already feeling relaxed. Begin by paying attention to how you're breathing while you're feeling tense. Then use the mind and body connection to affect the change. Changing your mind reflects change in your body, and vice versa. Conscious breathing is a power-tool for re-programming your nervous system.

Mouth breathing isn't the only action that can be connected to excessive muscle tension. It's possible to determine the information that you're programming into your nervous system by observing your breathing patterns. Even though your mind and body work together and affect each other, remember that you, the user, are in control. Your actions will always be the result of your thoughts. Have you noticed yourself recurrently doing anything on the following list?

a) Yawning
b) Sighing frequently
c) Huffing when irritated
d) Holding your breath when concentrating
e) Raising your shoulders when taking in a deep breath

All of the above could be signs of stress underlying the cause of muscle tension imbalance. You can train yourself to notice when you're expressing your breath in any of these ways. Pay attention to what you were thinking directly before you noticed the breathing expression. Then consciously take in a deep breath, and release it slowly out through your nose. Think of the word 'relax' as you breathe out. Consciously train your breathing to respond to positive thoughts, rather than unconsciously reacting to your negative ones.

It may help you with this process to understand the physical mechanics of breathing. Your diaphragm, the 'breathing muscle', is a large parachute shaped muscle that attaches to your ribs, chest, spine, and abdominal cavity. When you take a breath in it feels as if you're drawing air into your lungs, but this isn't actually the case. Inhaling is the autonomic act of flexing the diaphragm and intercostal muscles, which expands the ribs. Air is then 'pushed' into your empty lungs due to the greater pressure of the air on the outside of your body.

The act of exhaling brings the diaphragm back up to its starting position. This forces the air out of the lungs and creates a vacuum. The volume of your in-breath is therefore determined by the completeness of your out-breathe. Fight-or-flight response can interfere with this completeness, by incorporating the muscles of your chest and neck. Unlike the diaphragm, these muscles are voluntary when it comes to respiration. Breathing with your neck and chest, rather than your diaphragm, is like driving your car on only half a tank of fuel. When you're working with less than full capacity – you're much more likely to run out of gas!

The following is an exercise that you can use to practice breathing fully with your diaphragm and intercostal muscles. You're not actually making the diaphragm work. This muscle is autonomic and will work whether you think about it or not. Obviously this is the case, or you'd have died the first time you fell asleep! The practice is about getting the other muscles to relax, and to get out of the way.

BELLY BREATHING

Please read through the entire exercise before beginning to practice. Practice facing a mirror until you can take in a deep breath without raising your shoulders at the same time.

ONE: Sit in a comfortable chair and begin to relax.
TWO: Place your hands on your belly, one above and one below your navel.
THREE: Take a deep breath in for the count of three (if three is too long then begin with two).
FOUR: Imagine pushing your navel out and down towards your knees as you breathe in.
FIVE: Breathe out to the count of four (if four is too long then begin with three).
SIX: Think of the word 'relax', and focus on letting go of tension as you breathe out.
SEVEN: Repeat the above exercise within your comfort level.

Provided that you don't feel any dizziness or discomfort while practicing belly breathing, begin with ten repetitions. Build up to a count of twenty-one per session. If you find it uncomfortable at first, then begin with two repetitions and gradually increase from there at your own pace.

Once you've mastered the practice of belly-breathing with comfort, you'll have taken a major step towards stretching your body with ease.

ONE POSITION SYNDROME

Many occupations in the world today call for long periods of sitting, standing, or bending. Even hobbies such as knitting, gardening, and reading can present the same problem. Resting the buttocks on a chair, bench or couch is considered to be perfectly normal now in our society. But this prolonged sitting is far from natural behavior, and it certainly isn't beneficial for the body.

One position syndrome' is exacerbated by furniture being bought and sold as generic. How can one particular armchair correctly support a six-foot, two hundred and thirty pound man, and also correctly support a five-foot, one hundred and ten pound woman? The answer is quite simple of course - it can't. A particular chair will have the lumbar and neck support in the right place for a particular height and size of person. That same chair however, will be all wrong for someone of a different height and size.

When a chair is supporting you properly, you'll be able to relax completely. When a chair is not supporting you properly, certain muscles will tighten up to hold you in position. This creates an incorrect muscle pattern, making it difficult for you to relax. Over time the muscles that are supporting you become chronically short. The opposing muscles become chronically lengthened and weak. The pain that accompanies this poor posture creeps up on you insidiously; until one day you feel that first twinge.

Ironically you probably won't feel that twinge while sitting at your desk, or on the couch. That first pinch of pain will be felt when you bend down to pick something up, or reach up to an overhead shelf. You'll feel the pain when you least expect to feel it. When you make a move that requires those chronically tight muscles to stretch out, and they don't comply. Your more flexible muscles will take the strain, and in these muscles you'll feel the first twinge.

Chronic pain is not necessarily felt in the muscles that are at root cause of the problem. 'One position syndrome' is exacerbated because of this misdirection. You may well be reacting to the pain signals that your body's sending to you, but you're stretching the wrong area in response. An example of this would be back pain caused by sitting at a computer all day. Stretching the weak and lengthened muscles of your back will only lead to more tension. You'll need to stretch the tight and shortened muscles of your chest to create balance and lasting relief.

Correcting the way that you're sitting in the first place is the way to release your pain chain from the source. This doesn't need to require a great deal of your time or your money. You don't necessarily need to buy a new chair, or pay for fancy ergonomic gadgets. With the right kind of knowhow, and a little awareness, you can do your own ergonomic assessment. Then make the necessary adjustments based on what you discover. You just might be kicking yourself under the desk, when you realize that you're the one that's been adding links to your chain!

First off, check that both feet (heels and toes) are fully supported, with your thighs parallel to the ground. If your feet don't reach the ground and you can't adjust your chair, then use a footstool or a telephone book. When your legs hang over the edge of the chair, their weight will pull on your pelvis and cause your lower back to tighten up. Additionally, sitting with your feet tucked back underneath and behind you is an attempt to balance that lower back tension. Have your feet correctly supported to allow your lower back muscles to relax.

Sit with the lumber support in your lumbar area, not against your buttocks or the back of your shoulders. This is perhaps the trickiest one of all to get right. If the lumbar support is too high, or too low, when you allow yourself to relax you'll slump forward. If the lumbar support is too bulky it'll feel uncomfortable, and may push you forward in the seat. Try different cushions; roll up a towel, or use a pillow to find the perfect fit for your body. When you support your lumbar area in the correct place, your back will thank you for it.

Sit upright with the computer screen, and your paper-stand at eye level. Holding your head tilted up, or down for long periods can cause excessive tension in your neck and upper back. Lift your chest, and position your screen and your paperwork where you can look at them without tilting your chin. To raise your screen or paperwork to eyelevel, you can purchase a stand from an office supply store. Alternatively, you can use a pile of books if you don't want to venture out to the store.

Some workstations are set up with two desks forming an 'L' shape. One desk is for a computer, and the other one is usually used as a writing table. If this applies to you, then you need to be sitting in a swivel chair. Avoid at all costs having your chair facing one desk, and your body turning at the waist to work at the other. Sitting in a swivel chair allows you to turn your entire body from one position to another. At all times have your knees directly facing the station that you're working at.

Sitting with your knees apart and your toes pointing out is a sure sign of tight hip muscles. Tight outer hips are a major cause of chronic lower back pain. In fact, Piriformis Syndrome is often misdiagnosed as sciatica, because the pain felt in the buttocks is similar. The Piriformis is a strong strap like muscle that attaches your thigh bone to your hip bone so to speak. It's responsible for laterally rotating your leg, and turning your foot out to the side.

A simple way to create a gentle stretch is to draw your knees together when you're sitting down. At the same time turn your feet to face forward, provided of course that this doesn't cause you any pain or discomfort. You could even hold your knees together with a soft belt while watching TV. This'll allow you to relax and still hold the correct position. Don't tie the belt with a knot though, just wrap it around your knees and hold it with your hand.

There'll be times when you just can't avoid sitting or standing in one position. If your job calls for it, then there's just not much you can do about it. Standing in line at the bank or store can be tedious, but now-a-days it's only to be expected. What you can avoid however, is developing one-position-syndrome. Make your best effort to sit or stand correctly, and relax your shoulders. Adjust your workstation if necessary to maintain good posture. As the saying goes, "an ounce of prevention is worth a pound of cure!"

GRAVITY IS RELATIVE

There's no movement that you can make, asleep or awake, standing or sitting that isn't relative to gravity. When standing up straight, your COG (center of gravity) is a straight line running perpendicular to the ground. It runs up through the front of your ankle, and the middle of your knee, hip, shoulder, and ear.

Gravity pulls straight down, and there are no exceptions to this rule. When you lean forward, certain muscles will have to adjust to stop you from falling on your face! If your job requires you to stand for long periods of time, you probably won't be standing up straight for most of it. More than likely you'll be leaning over a counter, or frequently twisting or bending down.

My client Jimmy had been working as a grocery store clerk for over three years. He was suffering with chronic lower back pain. Jimmy had never even heard of the term 'center of gravity', let alone know how to find it. He wasn't thinking about his body at all when he was reaching for an item to swipe at the cash register.

The first step towards relief for Jimmy was to position his feet with the weight evenly distributed between them. The next step was for him to learn how to move correctly from the hips, with conscious awareness of his COG. Finally, I tailored a corrective stretching program for him to follow every day. After three weeks of correcting his posture and gentle stretching, Jimmy was finally able to cast off his chronic pain chain.

Just because you've had back pain for years, it doesn't mean that you have to continue to suffer with it. Just because nothing shows up on an MRI, it doesn't mean that you're a victim of some universal mystery. Find the cause of the problem, and break the chain for yourself. This can begin with some simple exercises that require nothing more than your conscious attention.

Teach yourself to stand with your weight evenly balanced between your feet. Do this deliberately whenever you possibly can. Do it consciously until it becomes unconscious. Be aware of your COG while you're standing in line at the store, talking to a friend in the street, using the ATM, or washing dishes. It's particularly important to balance your weight if your job calls for long periods on your feet. I've been standing correctly for so long now that to stand any other way would feel uncomfortable.

Center of gravity is equally important when you're sitting down. Being aware of your COG can help you to release unnecessary tension. If your body isn't being supported properly in your seat, when you try to relax you'll slouch forward. Gravity would pull out of the chair unless you tensed specific muscles to prevent it. Gravity pulls straight down, always and without exceptions.

I can't talk about your center of gravity without a mention here of high-heeled shoes. There appears to be some controversy as to who first invented this type of unnatural and torturous footwear. Apparently they were commonly used in the fifteen hundreds; although high-heeled shoes in some form or another have been recorded in cultures dating back much further. Prior to the French Revolution, both men and women were tottering around on these stilts. At some point in the past couple of hundred years men wised up!

Women today are still venturing out on three and four inch spikes. Raising your heels that high above your toes shifts your center of gravity forward. This causes your calf and back muscles to tighten up in response. The problems caused by this happening aren't always felt immediately; but they will be eventually. Is following this fashion really worth creating a chronic pain chain?

Women don't wear high-heeled shoes for the benefit of other women. They do so presumably to attract, or keep, a mate. Why else would she want to create this particular 'look'? Is a woman less attractive with her heels firmly resting on the ground? If nature deemed high-heels to be necessary for sexual attraction, then women would have bony protrusions lifting them up onto the balls of their feet.

I can't say that I never wear 'heels', because I do. They're not very high, and I only wear them for special occasions. If any pair of shoes in my closet caused me to utter the sentence, "my feet are killing me," they'd be dumped unceremoniously at the thrift shop. Could traipsing around in your fashionable stilts be causing your lower back pain – absolutely! Do you think it's worth it? Only you can answer that question.

WATCHING TV SYNDROME

Staring at a television is a regular pastime for much of the population today. People are watching TV for hours at a time, and for a multitude of reasons. After a hard day's work do you sit in front of the box attempting to relax? TV time could indeed be a great way to unwind, depending on a couple of considerations. The first is the position in which you're sitting. How you support your body is always going to be important of course.

My clients are often aware of the need to have their computer screen at eye level. Ironically though, I've discovered that it rarely occurs to them to apply the same rule to the television. Watching the box in any one of the following positions could be causing your chronic pain:

a) Lying on your stomach looking up at the television
b) Lying or sitting with your head turned to the side to see the screen
c) Sitting and looking up at a TV hanging above eye level on the wall

To avoid causing 'watching TV syndrome', position your set directly in front of you, and at eye level. It's no less important than correct positioning of your computer screen. It may actually be even more important depending on the time ratio. Many people spend more time watching their favorite shows, than they do working or playing on a computer. TV time can often be less relaxing, than it is adding links to a chronic pain chain.

The second consideration is the less obvious one, and is often not even considered at all. The tension in your body is affected not only by how you're sitting, but by what you're watching! Your body is responding to your thoughts; not the physical circumstances around you. When you're watching a violent scene on the screen, you may as well be there yourself.

Thrillers are called that for a reason; they're designed to stimulate fear in the audience. The more gasps and screams a horror movie can generate, the more successful it's considered to be. You may not be a screamer, but if you're into fast paced adventure then you're body's ready for action too. These stimulating kind of movies and programs are fine once in a while. But causing your body to produce adrenalin on a regular basis can be harmful to your health.

Your nervous system responds to the information that you're feeding into it. It doesn't judge that information - but you do. Fear and excitement aren't the only emotional affects stimulated by watching television. Feelings of anger, indignation, and jealousy are just a few of many more feelings that lead to physical responses. Producing adrenalin can feel as if it's a natural expression of passion, particularly if it's in response to a personal or political belief. If this sounds like you, then ask yourself this question, "Is doing this to myself helping me to relax?"

Sitting with poor posture can lead to 'watching TV syndrome'. Heavy dramas, political discussions, and so-called 'reality shows', can also just as easily lead to painful tension. By all means enjoy a good movie and your favorite shows for entertainment. I love a stimulating adventure flick myself. But lighten up, or at least wise up. No matter which station you may be watching, the only program that really matters is the one you're producing in your own life!

PERFECT POSTURE

Your posture is the result of muscle tension responding to your thoughts. A poised and confident person stands tall, chest up, and shoulders relaxed. This is what we call 'good posture'. Thoughts of uncertainty, fear, and indecisiveness can lead to the protective posture of slouching. A frightened animal will attempt to protect its most vulnerable areas. You're doing the same thing when you curl your shoulders around, and fold your arms across your solar plexus.

Poise creates good posture that leads to personal power; a pretty simple equation. No one is likely to think of slouching as the path to self-empowerment. Why then is good posture so rarely observed, and round shoulders positively common? The answer to this question begins with taking a closer look at the meaning of confidence. People with good posture have a positive air of confidence and clarity about them.

When you're clear about what you're doing, and confident that you know how to do it, then you're poised for success. To feel confident you must first be aware of what you really want to achieve, which may not be as simple as it sounds. The second step to confidence is even more important. The second step is believing that you deserve to have the experience. Knowing what you want is useless if you don't believe that you deserve to have it.

Living long term in disagreement with someone such as a boss, or life partner, can knock your confidence for six. Disagreements can lead to a fear of aggression and confrontation. It's not conflicting views themselves that cause confrontations though. Aggression arises when one person is attempting to force his or her viewpoint on another. Dreading confrontation is not the fear of defending your opinion; it's the fear that you won't be able to.

Always strive to be clear about what you believe at any given moment. Allow yourself to change your mind when more information is presented. Trust in your ability to make your own choices. Don't be quick to blame the other person for causing the conflict. Ask yourself if it's really necessary for your opinion to be understood by someone else. When your intentions are always to peacefully resolve rather than to debate, confrontation no longer promotes fear in your life.

The personal power part of the equation is achieved by realizing that your thoughts are causing all of your life experiences. Whether you're standing tall or slouching forward, your body is simply acting in response to those thoughts. Perfect posture begins with taking full responsibility for what you're doing, and why you're doing it. The next step is to release the excessive tension caused by your previous thoughts, and restore a healthy balance.

Being aware of how you're sitting and standing all day can be an arduous task. Ironically, chronic pain relief is not always incentive enough to do this. For many people there's a much greater incentive – the realization that it can be the quickest weight loss program ever! Standing up straight can make you look as if you've just lost ten pounds. And that's not all… making the effort to sit or stand up straight could do all of the following for you:

1. Make you look thinner
2. Raise your energy level
3. Strengthen the muscles of your back

4. Improve your ability to breathe properly

5. Improve your agility and range of motion

You can achieve all of the items on the above list without even breaking a sweat. The following is an exercise that I teach to my clients' to help them improve their overall posture. The only equipment required is a mirror, and it takes just a couple of minutes to complete.

> ONE: Stand in front of a mirror.
> TWO: Place your hand on your chest; it doesn't matter which hand.
> THREE: Keep your eyes on your shoulders in the mirror.
> FOUR: Lift your chest (ribcage, not shoulders) and stand up straight.
> FIVE: Notice if you also lifted your shoulders up as you lifted your chest.
> SIX: Relax, and then repeat the chest lift again, this time without raising your shoulders.
> SEVEN: Imagine pulling your scapula down your back, and putting them in the pockets of your trousers.
> EIGHT: Gently press your navel back against your spine, so that you don't pop your hips forward.
> NINE: Hold your corrected posture with shoulders relaxed for thirty seconds, breathing normally.
> TEN: Relax and release the position.

It may take practice for you to lift your chest and stand up straight without lifting your shoulders at the same time. Another habit that can be difficult to let go of is popping your hips forward when you straighten up. This is why I suggest doing the exercise facing a mirror. Being able to observe your body as you move will help you to gain greater awareness. Eventually you'll be able to feel the position of your body without needing visual aids.

Even though the above exercise only takes a couple of minutes, it isn't crucial for creating good posture. It isn't essential to do any kind of structured exercise at all. It is necessary however, to pay attention to how you're sitting and standing on a moment to moment basis. You need to be prepared to make the effort if you're going to create better habits. There's no such thing as not having enough time to restore your good posture. If you have the time to slump, then you have time to sit up straight.

Now of course the environment of your work and home is going to influence how you sit and stand. These factors are still going to be trumped by the habits that you've formed along the way. Correcting your posture will probably be difficult at first, like going to the gym after years of being a couch potato. Begin by sitting up straight for just a couple of minutes at a time, four times an hour for a week. Then increase to five minutes at a time, three times an hour for a week, and so on.

Gradually your back muscles will shorten and strengthen, and your chest muscles will relax and stretch out. It'll get easier each day to sit up correctly. In fact, with practice it will begin to feel uncomfortable to sit slumped over again. What better motivation can you have for perfecting your posture, than the list of benefits I previously gave you? Here is a reminder of what standing tall could do for you:

1. Makes you look thinner
2. Raises your energy level
3. Strengthens the muscles of your back
4. Improves your ability to breathe properly
5. Improves your agility and range of motion

It's possible that your poor stance is aggravated by an exceptionally rounded upper spine, clinically known as excessive kyphosis. This is relatively common; I have it myself. Maintaining strong and flexible back muscles helps to prevent this condition from deteriorating. If I hadn't started making the effort years ago to stand up straight, I'd be looking like the Hunch Back of Notre Dame by now!

Whatever the underlying cause of your poor posture, be it congenital, habitual, or both, you can take action to do something about it. You may not be experiencing any pain yet, but that doesn't mean that you won't be eventually. There's that old saying again, "an ounce of prevention is worth a pound of cure." If you don't stand up for yourself today, it'll be a lot tougher to achieve in the future. And remember, your posture isn't something that you have; your posture is a reflection of who you are!

POSITIONING YOUR PELVIS

Without a shadow of a doubt there's one talent that Elvis Presley had truly mastered. No I'm not talking about singing; I'm talking about gyrating his pelvis! Can you do what Elvis did with such finesse? If not, then you probably have an imbalance in the muscle tension of your hips, back, and thighs.

Whether you're sitting, standing, lunging, squatting, or bending, the position of your pelvis will reveal any muscle tension imbalance. When the muscles of your hips and back are working in harmony, your pelvis will be level when you're standing up. This means that it'll be parallel with the floor beneath you. Both your pelvis and your chest will be parallel with the wall that you're facing. Last but not least, the bony crowns of your pelvis will be facing upwards.

Muscle tension that's out of balance due to your behavior can adversely affect your joints, and your range of motion. If the top of one hipbone is sitting lower than the other, a tight piriformis muscle could be the culprit. It's not the only possible cause though. Structural abnormalities can also affect the tension of skeletal muscles, pulling the pelvis out of line.

One hip could appear to be lower than the other due to a congenital condition, such as scoliosis of the spine. Then there's the possibility of a degenerative process affecting the balance of muscle tension. Specific stretching and strengthening of muscle groups can help with these issues, once you know what you're dealing with. If you haven't already done so, get yourself checked out to be sure.

Once you have the go-ahead to exercise freely from your physician, the lunge position is often recommended to stretch tight hip flexors. Your hip flexor muscles raise your knees, lifting your feet up off the ground. While standing in a lunge position, take a look at the level of your hips. If the hip of the back leg sits further back than the hip of the front leg, you could be dealing with a tight psoas muscle.

The psoas is a powerful muscle that attaches at one end to the vertebrae of your lower back. The other end connects at the top of your thigh; one on each side. Long periods of sitting cause these thick strap-like muscles to shorten. Over time they lock in that shortened position, stressing your lower back when you're standing up. At this point you may no longer be able to effectively isolate and stretch the psoas muscles by means of lunging. This is particularly the case if the hip of your back leg not only sits further back, but also dips down below the front hip.

When the psoas muscles of both hips are chronically tight from sitting, they also pull the pelvis forward when you stand up. A forward pelvic tilt is what's commonly known as 'swayback'. I notice swayback more often in women, but not by any means exclusively. Tight hip-flexors, along with weak back and abdominal muscles, are a major cause of swayback. And sway back is a major cause of chronic lower back pain.

To improve the effectiveness of your lunge, consciously correct the position of your pelvis. Tuck your tailbone under, and pull your navel back toward your spine. This will help you to target the deep seated psoas muscle. You may feel a gentle stretch in the small of your back, as well as the front of your thigh. However, if you experience pain, pinching, burning, or any other uncomfortable sensation, you're to stop stretching immediately.

When hip flexor muscles have firmly adopted a shortened position, it may not be possible for you to consciously correct your lunge. Another gentle stretch for the difficult to isolate psoas can be performed lying on your back.

Lie on the bed with your legs bent at the knees and dangling over the end. Bring your left knee up to your chest with your hands, and press your navel down towards your spine. Relax the right leg, and allow the weight of the leg to create a gentle stretch. You should be feeling this stretch closer to where the muscle attaches in the front of your right thigh.

Muscles that have already been out of balance for a while though may be stubbornly tight. This can cause a feeling of pulling and discomfort in your lower back. If this is the case, then begin with the extended leg supported on the bed, rather than hanging over the end. It's possible that even this stretch may be too uncomfortable for you in the beginning. It's okay to place a pillow under the knee of your extended leg to help you to relax.

Standing with good posture is practically impossible to achieve with one or both shortened psoas muscles. Stretching alone isn't going to fix this problem though. It's important to maintain both the strength, as well as the flexibility of these vital hip and pelvis flexors. Sitting for long periods of time upsets the delicate balance between strength and flexibility. It's not when you're sitting that you'll feel the fallout for this though. You'll feel that lower back pain when you get up to do something else!

Even when you're physically fit, there can be times when back pain can get your goat while you're walking. If this is happening to you, try pushing off the back foot as you're stepping forward. At the same time, consciously lift your front knee a little higher. It may feel rather like you're marching. If this relieves the symptoms, go ahead and add standing knee raises to your exercise routine. Alternating knee raises (raising your knee as high as you can without leaning forward) will strengthen your hip flexors.

Another safe and easy exercise for balancing strength with flexibility is the 'pelvic tilt'. This simple movement will involve not only the hip flexors, but the muscles of your abdomen and back. This is particularly useful for a gentle approach to correcting swayback. Pelvic tilting against the wall calls for equal effort from the muscles of the upper back.

Performing the exercise lying on the ground is less challenging, and focuses more emphasis on the hip flexors and the abdominal muscles.

Stand with your buttocks and the back of your shoulders up against a wall. Slide your hands into the gap behind your lower back, at the level of your navel. Now take your hands back out again. Next, press your navel back against your spine, until there's no longer a gap for you to slip your hands into. Don't allow yourself to bend forward. Keep both shoulders and your buttocks in contact with the wall throughout. Hold for three deep breaths as you perform this simple pelvic tilt, and then relax. Repeat ten times.

To perform the pelvic tilt lying on your back, bend your knees with your feet a shoulder width apart. Slide your hands into the gap under your lower back. Next, remove your hands and then press your navel down against the ground. You should no longer be able to get your hands under your lower back. Feel the roll of the pelvis, as you perform the pelvic tilt exercises. To increase the intensity of the exercise, lift your feet a couple of inches up off the ground. For maximum challenge, place the soles of your feet together and let your knees fall apart. There's to be no pain or discomfort felt at any time.

Corrective exercising is an important part of creating a balanced and blissful body. No matter how much effort you put into it though, you'll always fall short of success if you don't address the underlying causes. Sitting for long periods without stretching is a well-recognized cause of lower back pain. Ironically, I've discovered that this knowledge is frequently ignored, despite the painful consequences.

Spending your time sitting down is not the only cause of lower back pain. You may have many other habits that are equally culpable. To make the most of your corrective exercises, you'll need to make the effort to create better habits. You can break the chronic pain chain at the source by always observing the following:

1. Sit upright with correct lumbar support.

2. Have both feet properly supported when sitting.
3. Sit with your thighs parallel to the ground beneath you.
4. Stand with your weight evenly distributed on both feet.
5. Whether sitting or standing, walk and stretch every twenty minutes.

How long it takes you to break your chain will be determined by how much effort you're prepared to put into it. Knowledge is useless to you without the motivation to put it into action. After all, it's your back that's up against the wall!

STRETCHING BLIND SPOTS

You have a natural reflex to stretch out the muscles of your body every day; just like a cat waking up from a nap. However, it's quite likely that unlike your furry companion, you've learned to ignore this reflex. Doing 'what comes naturally' is frequently being replaced today with a 'stretching routine'. After a long day of sitting or standing mostly in one spot, a string of preconceived stretches are performed either before, or after exercising. And in some cases, without the exercising part at all.

Throwing down a mat and stretching out your tightly wound-up body, is better than no stretching at all. However, stretching correctly may not be quite what you think it is. Are you following the same routine every time, or are you mixing it up with a variety? Even if you stretch religiously day after day, stretching some muscles while neglecting others will perpetuate muscle tension imbalance. You could be simply stretching out the links of your own chronic pain chain!

While I was teaching a yoga class one day, I noticed something that I found interesting about stretching. The students were unconsciously holding postures longer on one side, than they were holding on the other. More interesting still, I observed that it wasn't the tighter side that was being stretched for longer periods.

Following that observation, I was disconcerted to realize that I had that very same blind spot! I was demonstrating poses to the right side first, because it was easier for me to relax while explaining to the students. Then I'd practically skip going to the left side altogether. Instead I'd walk around the room correcting the posture of the students. Shedding light on that blind spot opened my eyes to the importance of symmetry. Equal time needs to be dedicated to each side when practicing poses with a left and a right hand face.

Over the years I've worked with incredibly fit body builders and athletes. Unfortunately, physical prowess is no guarantee that a chronic pain chain isn't being forged. Habitually stretching certain muscles, while neglecting others, is a fast track to suffering. No matter what your fitness level, the natural urge to stretch cannot be completely suppressed. It can however, be confused.

Where you feel tightness, aching, or discomfort isn't always where you'll find the source of the problem. For example, the cause of aching on the right side of your neck could be due to chronically tight and shortened muscles on the left. The longer muscles on the right are trying to contract to restore balance, but the opposing muscles are refusing to cooperate. Even though discomfort is being felt on the right side, continually stretching the longer muscles will only exacerbate the problem. The way to break this particular chain is to address the cause of shortened muscles on the left-hand side of the neck.

It's not always possible to visually locate a tight problem muscle. Particularly if it happens to be a deep hip flexor, as I previously mentioned. There are times however, when a tight area is quite apparent, but you just haven't noticed it yet. So stand in front of a mirror, and take a good look at your outline. Is the line between your earlobes and your collarbone equal on both sides? Are your shoulders level? Is there equal length on both sides between your armpit and the crown of your hip?

It may be easier than you realized to see which, if any, of your tight muscles have become chronically short. If you determine that this actually is the case for you, the next step is to figure out why it happened. It's quite possible that you're unconsciously perpetuating the problem. Take a look at the situations listed below. Could one or more of them be concealing a stretching realization blind spot for you?

a) An injury caused you to avoid certain movements in the past. Even though the injury has since healed, the resulting muscle tension remains out of balance.

b) You're sitting, standing, moving, or sleeping in a poorly supported position.

c) You have a congenital abnormality, such as a short tendon, calcification around a joint, or scoliosis.

You may be avoiding a certain stretch or movement, because it causes you to feel acute pain. Acute pain could be a sign that something more serious is going on. This kind of situation calls for a consultation with a physician. Stretching is never to be the cause of acute pain. The purpose of stretching is to balance muscle tension, and to relieve any associated chronic discomfort.

Let's say that your physician has determined that you don't have any kind illness or injury. Yet still, when you attempt to stretch out the pain is sharp and extremely uncomfortable. In a scenario like this it may be the way that you're stretching that's causing the problem. The following is a list of important points to remember when you're performing any kind of stretch:

1. Sit, stand, or lie in a stable position that allows you to relax completely before you begin to stretch.

2. Take in a deep breath, and stretch as you're breathing out.

3. Consciously relax and allow the muscles to lengthen. Attempting to force a stretch will only risk tearing muscle fibers, and could result in injury.

4. Don't 'bounce' to make the stretch go further. Bouncing is a habit that causes the nervous system to keep 'firing' into the muscle. This could also lead to an injury.

5. When stretching first to the left, and then to the right, always stretch to both sides for an equal length of time.

6. If you're stretching in a group class, focus only on yourself. Pay no attention to what other people are doing.

When it's done consciously and correctly, stretching is an important part of improving flexibility. When you're stretching with a realization blind spot however, it could be causing your pain rather than fixing it. A safe and effective stretching routine will contain all of the following:

1. Knowledge of any congenital spine, joint, or ligament issues that need to be considered.

2. Full awareness of the ROM (range of motion) for each of your joints. For example, can you raise both arms overhead equally, or does one fall short of the other?

3. A well-balanced routine will also contain a wide variety of stretches. It'll be designed to correctly address all of your skeletal muscles.

ROM (RANGE OF MOTION)

Your ROM (range of motion) refers to how far you can move around a joint. For example, the ROM of your left arm will be the following:

1. How high you can comfortably lift your arm overhead, reaching first out front, and then from the side of your body.
2. How far you can reach your arm straight out behind you with your palm facing upwards. There's to be no pinching, burning, or any other kind of pain.
3. How far you can slide your left thumb up your back between your shoulder blades.
4. How high you can lift your elbow with your hand resting on your shoulder; to the front, and then to the side.
5. How far you can stretch your arm across your chest, without turning or moving your body.

These few movements will give you a good assessment of the ROM of your left shoulder. Repeat the assessment on the right side, and then compare the ROM of the left shoulder to the right one. This'll provide you with necessary information for creating an effective stretching routine. Flexibility isn't about stretching as far as you can go. Flexibility is about balancing stretch and strength to create optimum ROM in all joints.

When there's too much stretch in muscles without the required opposing strength, the joint becomes unstable. This is evident in someone who's always dislocating, or 'popping out' his or her shoulder. An unstable joint can result from damage to one or more of the ligaments that attach the muscles to the bones. In a case like this, optimum flexibility will require strengthening certain muscles, rather than just stretching them.

It isn't necessary to know the names of your muscles to have a great stretching routine. It is necessary however to know the ROM of your joints. If you're experiencing pain when you move a specific joint, get a physician to take a look before you start doing your self-assessment.

It's pretty simple to determine the safe ROM for each specific joint. Just ask yourself this question, "would this particular movement be one that I would ever make in my everyday life?" For example, it would never be necessary or practical for you to put your leg behind your head. You probably would however, find it necessary at times to reach your arm out in front of you.

It's not just ROM that determines if a movement is practical though, it's also the accompanying strength. When I personally need to lift a box down from a high shelf, I ask myself both of these questions: "Can I reach the box safely without needing a step? Am I certain that I have the strength to lift it down without hurting myself?"

You can ask yourself the same two questions, but be honest about it. It could be the difference between hurting yourself, or not. Lifting a heavy object either up, or down without adequate strength and ROM is a major cause of injury. If you're in any doubt – don't do it. Ignorance and stubbornness could land you in the hospital!

Every move you make involves more than just one joint. Lifting something safely requires knowledge of the strength and ROM of your shoulders. You'll also need to know where you stand with your wrists, elbows, spine, knees, and ankles too. Try lifting anything up from the ground, or down off of a shelf, without flexing all of these joints.

Take the time to get to know your own strengths and limitations. It's the best way to prevent yourself from being the cause of your own pain. Keep in mind that no one is text book symmetrical. You're making many one-sided movements every day, probably without even giving it a thought. Driving, writing, playing sports, and answering the telephone are all asymmetrical movements. It's not necessary to create perfect physical symmetry; only to create adequately balanced ROM for your safety and comfort.

71

AGILITY

When I was a little girl I loved to cartwheel on the village green. Thanks to regular yoga practice, I'm still fit enough to do it today. Sadly, now that I'm all grown up, it would be inappropriate to have such unbridled fun! Not many adults maintain the level of flexibility that they had in childhood. Compounding this problem today, children themselves are suffering the effects of a sedentary lifestyle.

I doubt of course that it'll ever be necessary for you to cartwheel across your lawn. But there's a wide range of movements between playing active games and performing functional activities. No matter what age you are at the moment, losing your sprightliness can be a real pain. To determine your current level of agility, how many functions on the following list can you perform with ease?

1. Getting down and back up off the ground without leaning on something
2. Jumping up at least six inches off the ground
3. Squatting all the way down on your heels
4. Kneeling down on the floor
5. Bending over from the hips
6. Climbing stairs

To set your short term goal for agility, think about something that you want to achieve. For example, do you want to be able to reach up and change a light bulb by yourself? Use this goal to begin improving the balance and ROM necessary to achieve it. If you can already reach up with your left hand, but can barely lift your right hand above the shoulder, then focus on improving the ROM of your right shoulder.

Through my work with clients, I've discovered that limited ROM isn't due entirely to having weak or tight muscles. Limited movement can be due to the anticipation of feeling pain. Apart from being a 'realization blind spot', this also causes a catch 22. When you anticipate feeling pain, your muscles tighten in response to your thoughts. When your muscles tighten it makes it more difficult for you to move freely. Restricted movement causes discomfort, and your muscles tighten up even more.

To determine the true range of motion, take in a deep breath and completely relax before beginning to move. This may take some practice if you're used to a 'pain anticipation' reaction to movement. Use your breath to relax every step of the way. If you begin to feel pain, then stop at that point. Take in a deep slow breath, and consciously relax the muscles around the joint as you breathe out.

Pain caused by a 'pain anticipation' reaction will ease when you consciously stop anticipating it. Support your arm or leg if necessary in the extended position; this will help you to more easily relax. If the pain increases no matter what you do, you may have an unresolved injury. Increasing pain can also result from stressing the ligaments of an unstable joint. No matter what the cause, if the pain intensifies stop the exercise immediately. With practice you'll be able to eliminate any 'pain anticipation' reaction altogether, and find the true range of motion.

The goal of stretching is to create sufficient flexibility to perform your day to day activities. Being able to touch your toes may not be a useful goal in itself. Being able to pull your socks on and off however, is a whole other story. The purpose of stretching is to improve the balanced flexibility of your skeletal muscles. Balanced flexibility creates optimum, and safe 'range of motion' for the moveable joints of your body.

YOGA

In western society today, yoga has become practically synonymous with stretching. It's true to say that stretching is involved in practicing an asana (body posture). But to say that yoga is about stretching, is like saying that your car is about grocery shopping. Is driving to the store the purpose of your car, and the limit of what it can do for you? Of course not!

Stretching is just one aspect of ssana practice, and body postures are only one limb of yoga's eight limbed holistic science.

There are approximately eight hundred and forty thousand asanas, according to 'Yoga – The Science of Holistic Living', by Vivekananda Kendra Patrika. As I mentioned earlier, the most important asana of all is considered to be Savasana, or Corpse Pose. This position is traditionally practiced at the end of a group class. Savasana is considered to be practicing 'stillness in action'. You simply lie still on your back on the ground, and completely relax. Ironically, Corpse Pose is one of the most difficult for many people to achieve.

When the time comes for Savasana at the end of a class, I've witnessed students roll up their mats and leave. This has happened more often when the class is in a fitness club setting. Perhaps this is because yoga isn't primarily a practice of the body. Yoga is a practice of the Citta, which is a Sanskrit word meaning 'workings of the mind'. The atmosphere upon entering a gym, with the upbeat music and clashing of metal, is hardly conducive to a quiet and peaceful mind.

A yoga studio on the other hand, will attempt to create the whole 'yoga experience' from the moment you walk through the door. Relaxing music, soft lighting, inspiring plaques, and pastel colors, all encourage you to relax from the get go. No matter what the style, from vigorous Ashtanga to gentle Yin Yoga classes, genuine yoga practice will always end with Savasana, the Corpse Pose.

Practicing Corpse Pose several times a day has great potential benefits. The position is easy to achieve for just about everyone. It can be practiced on a firm bed, if getting down on the floor just isn't an option for you. With daily practice it can be a powerful tool for eliminating stressful tension from your life. To practice Savasana effectively, follow these guidelines:

ONE: Lie down on the ground. If getting on the ground isn't possible for you, then lie on the bed. Adopt a different position from the one in which you ordinarily sleep.

TWO: Ideally you won't need a pillow. If you do feel the need to support your head, use a small pillow, or a rolled up towel in the crook of your neck.

THREE: Place a pillow under your knees if you feel any discomfort in the small of your back.

FOUR: Let your arms rest loosely at your sides, and your legs slightly apart. It's okay to rest your hands on your body if you need to, but don't lace your fingers or cross your legs.

FIVE: Take deep slow belly breaths. Relax a different part of your body with each exhale. Begin with the muscles of your eyes.

If your mind is wandering and you find it difficult to focus, do one or more of the following:

a) Imagine yourself surrounded by swirling colored lights.

b) Count with your breathing: three counts in-breath and three counts out.

c) Count down slowly from ninety-nine, relaxing more and more with each number.

d) Imagine yourself in a field of flowers. See the blue sky above you, and feel the warm sun on your face.

Your muscles can remain tight and shortened even without your conscious awareness. Neck and shoulders are commonly the most difficult areas to relax, despite regular stretching. Having a realization blind spot about this can limit your range of motion. It can also lead to chronic pain and even injury. Savasana practice helps to relax and release this hindering tension from your body. Practicing Savasana can improve your flexibility without doing any stretching at all!

I reiterate here that where you're feeling pain isn't necessarily where the tightest problem muscles are located. This is why constantly stretching out the painful areas may not be bringing any lasting relief. The tightest problem muscles could be holding their position without relenting. Therefore the looser opposing muscles struggle to compensate and bring balance. The effort being made by the looser muscles to contract could be where you're feeling the chronic pain.

All yoga poses, but particularly the passive and meditative ones like Savasana, nurture awareness of muscle tension habits. All skeletal muscle contractions begin in the mind with a thought. Therefore mental awareness is the first step to relaxing unnecessary muscle tension. In Savasana you allow your body to completely surrender to the ground. There's no need for strength, balance, or flexibility to achieve this position. Any tension that you're still feeling in your body is therefore the result of chronically short muscles. You can now use your breath, the communicator between mind and body, to teach the nervous system to let go.

Improving flexibility isn't the only benefit of Savasana according to the book 'YOGA: Asanas, Pranayama, Mudras, Kriyas', by Vivekananda Kendra Prakashan, 12th edition 1999, page 45. In this book, published by Aye Yes Grafiks, Triplicane, Channai, India, it says:

> "BENEFITS: [of Savasana] One of the most powerful tools in controlling large number of diseases caused by tension, such as high blood pressure, and insomnia, etc. It is very helpful for calming down the mind leading to meditation."

The cultural poses of yoga such as Warrior, Side Twist, and Pigeon, are always performed twice: once for the left and once for the right. Other poses such as Bridge, Boat, and Plank call for a harmonious relationship between hips, back, and abdominals. The purpose of them all is to create muscular balance for holding and moving your body with ease.

Achieving the goal of muscular balance begins with mental awareness. If you're not aware of the purpose for practicing yoga poses, how can you be expected to reach the goal? To gain that greater mental awareness in your practice, ask yourself the following questions:

1. Hold long do I usually hold one pose in relationship to another?

2. Is holding a pose to the left, more or less comfortable than the same pose to the right?

3. Am I unconsciously holding my breath at any time during the practice?

4. Does consciously relaxing certain muscles make a pose easier to remain in?

5. Am I tightening my neck, or lifting my shoulders while holding a particular position?

There are so many 'styles' of yoga today that it can be difficult for the beginner to know where to start. There are many avenues available for practicing as well. You'll find classes at yoga studios, at gyms, and on home-use DVDs. Additionally, every instructor has his or her own personal background, personality, and teaching style.

Whether you're just starting out, or you're a seasoned Yogi, your safety should always be a primary consideration. It's wise to remember that just because you *can* do something, doesn't mean that you should. There are instructors that will guide a group class to perform head and shoulder stands. Even skilled and experienced teachers have injured themselves by practicing extreme inversions. Use your own common sense, and know when to say 'no'.

The original yoga postures were depicted thousands of years ago; long before western technology began crippling its people. In India today many children are still taught to practice yoga from an early age. It's also common for these people to sit crossed legged on the floor. In the western world, many children spend little time, if any, engaged in physical activity. They're also subjected to years of sitting on chairs. The resulting chronically tight muscles of the hips and back make many yoga postures difficult, if not practically impossible, to perform safely.

A pose such as the Shoulder Stand, places a great deal of pressure on the upper back and neck. You may be strong and flexible enough to get yourself into this position. If you choose to do so, keep your weight on your shoulders, and not on your neck. Creating a right-angle between your neck and your body places undue stress on your spine, and serves no purpose. When do you ever need to put your head into that position? No matter what your instructor tells you, if you're ever in doubt about the safety of a pose - don't do it!

Never force your neck into a sharp angle. The pressure applied to the nerves and blood vessels can cause injury, and even a stroke. Yoga is about uniting your mind, body, and spirit; it's not about pushing yourself to your physical limits. With wisdom and some commonsense, yoga practice is an excellent way to follow a painless path.

CHOOSING A YOGA STUDIO

Ask the studio owner if they follow a particular style there, or if there's a variety available. Having a variety of styles has its advantages. It gives you more opportunity to find out what will work well for your particular likes and needs. Also, don't just assume that the instructors are fully trained and experienced. Ask about their backgrounds and qualifications. You can often find this information on the studio website, so check there first.

Don't be afraid to ask for a description of a class with a particular name, such as: Yoga Pump, Hot Yoga, or Yogalates. Find out what to expect before you join in the class. Intensity can range from slow and gentle, to a heart pumping work out! Additionally, even a gentle class can be physically exhausting; particularly when the room temperature is about a hundred degrees Fahrenheit!

Most studios offer classes at a variety of days and time slots. If possible choose a time that's likely to be a smaller class. Midmornings and midafternoons are traditionally difficult classes to fill. Evenings after work are usually of course the most heavily populated. In a smaller class the instructor will be able to devote more attention to each student attending. In the beginning this could be an advantage for you.

Find out if you can take a free class, and then take it at the time you're most likely to be going to the studio. During the class, notice if the instructor demonstrates modifications for challenging poses. If the instructor is teaching with her back to you, you might want to run for the door. She won't see you leaving anyway! Mind you, it's becoming popular today for yoga studios to install mirrors on the wall. Use your discretion if this is the case; pay attention as to whether the instructor is watching the class in the mirror, or not.

Did the instructor encourage you to focus on your own body? Yoga isn't a competition sport. Trying to go as far as the next guy is a major cause of injury in a group class. You may be practicing as part of a group, but yoga is still a personal journey. Even the most experienced instructor can't watch every student all of the time. He or she should be reinforcing for you throughout that you're to always pay attention to the feedback from your body.

Perhaps you've already attended a class at a yoga studio, and your first experience wasn't a good one. Please don't write off yoga practice altogether based on that one time. There are so many great instructors out there, and so many ways to benefit from this time tested and proven science. I urge you to keep searching, until you find the right fit for your needs.

YOGA CLASSES AT THE GYM

There can be several issues to overcome when yoga classes are offered in a gym setting. Instructors will often crank the music up loud, then use headsets with speakers for their voices to be heard. Even above the super loud music, it's still possible to hear the thumping and banging of folks working out next door. The room is also often the same cold temperature as the rest of the gym.

A gym will usually offer a variety of dance and exercise classes in addition to yoga. There may only be one style or intensity level available for you to choose from. Classes are often scheduled back-to-back, with little to none change-over time. If there was an exercise class in the room directly before, the sweaty smell in there can be quite unpleasant. Last but not least, a yoga class in a gym usually has no size restrictions. I had forty-seven people crammed in a room one time!

There's always a Yin to the Yang though; a balance of pros and cons. Group classes are often included in the monthly gym membership fee. This is a big bonus for the financially challenged. Despite the drawbacks to the gym setting, there are still some great instructors teaching classes in these places. At least I think so, because I'm one of them! And after all, yoga is a practice of the mind. Being at peace with outside circumstances, no matter what they may be, is a part of the practice.

HOME USE YOGA DVD'S

If you're physically fit and not experiencing chronic pain, then the home use DVD may appear to be a good fit for you. The problem is that no matter how good the instructor may be, he or she can't see you following along. Being physically fit may not be enough to make sure that you're practicing correctly. If you have excessive muscle tension or poor posture, you'll be practicing yoga following your own incorrect patterns. You won't be able to tell if you're practicing correctly or not; and there'll be no one there to help you.

It may benefit you to take a couple of live classes before you start a home practice with a DVD. Mind you, if the classes are large you may still not get the attention that you need. It might be more useful to get an instructor to go over the DVD with you at home, before you practice with it by yourself. It's an extra financial investment that you may not be prepared to make. Consider though that hurting yourself could turn out to be a much greater financial drain.

At the very least, employ what you've learned here about how to use your breath. Stretch with awareness, and pay attention to what you're feeling in your body at all times. Don't try to push past your comfort level. If you doubt that you can perform a pose safely – don't even try it! There are many and varied DVD's out there showing you how to practice yoga. Look for one that's made especially for beginners. It wouldn't hurt if it was also specifically for back health too.

WORKING IT OUT

Every person that makes the effort to work out, whether at home or at the gym, has a personal reason in mind. No matter what the motivation, that reason is likely to fall into one of five categories. Each individual is probably trying to achieve one or more of the following:

> Lose weight
> Relieve stress
> Look and feel better
> Avoid or reverse a health issue
> Increase strength and endurance

If you're trying to de-stress by working out, or by taking physically demanding classes, there's something you need to consider. Stress causes an elevated heart rate and chronic muscle tension, which in turn can lead to health issues. According to the Mayo Clinic, common physical effects of stress include: headache, muscles tension or pain, chest pain, fatigue, change in sex drive, stomach upset, and sleep problems. Of course they recommend that if you're experiencing chest pain with shortness of breath you seek medical attention immediately.

A physically demanding workout raises the heart rate and adds additional tension to the skeletal muscles. Working-out this way may not be the best choice for you, when stress-relief is your goal. If you haven't already done so, check-up with your physician to eliminate any underlying medical problems. Then consult with a fitness professional to create a safe and effective routine. If working with a professional just isn't feasible for you, then consider yoga or tai chi, over a cardio-blast class or pumping iron.

WORKING WITH A PERSONAL TRAINER

Personal trainers, or fitness coaches as they're sometimes referred to, aren't required to be licensed in the USA. There are no national or state regulations that they have to follow, or exams that they have to take. There are however, a couple of hundred fitness organizations offering a variety of certifications. A handful of these organizations are considered to be top-notch, and some are not so reputable.

In my experience, the quality of the training is only one aspect of what makes an exceptional personal trainer. Another important consideration is the motivation for getting into the field in the first place. Many personal trainers have college degrees, but no experience. Many trainers are self-taught, but have no formal education at all. There's no guarantee either way that you're working with a trainer that's dedicated to achieving your goals.

Find out everything you can about your prospective trainer before you sign. What other skills or experience does he or she have? Your goals may be to lose weight and to improve agility. Your trainer may be more interested and experienced in body building. Don't be afraid to ask questions to find the right fit for your needs. The following are examples of what you might want to know about a personal trainer, before you commit to a program.

Is the trainer certified with an accredited organization?

Certification with an accredited organization isn't required to work as a personal trainer, but it's a good way to add credibility. I have ACSM (American College of Sports Medicine) certification. I found the academic training to be very thorough. The physical training part left a lot to be desired though. Fortunately, I already had years of experience in the field before I took the certification course.

There are several organizations offering personal training certifications that are accredited through NCCA (National Commission for Certification Agencies). If you want to check out a particular organization visit the website for NCCA: www.credentialingexcellence.org.

Is the trainer experienced working with a variety of equipment?

A personal trainer who only knows how to use one type of equipment is going to be limited. The same goes for a trainer that prefers to only use one type, such as machines. Equipment is not actually necessary at all for a good trainer to do his or her job. However, having a working knowledge of everything from Kettle Bells to Bosu balls, demonstrates an ability to challenge the client in a variety of ways.

Personal training sessions aren't cheap. You want to learn as much as you can from your trainer, and to be challenged and motivated. What you learn during your program can benefit you for the rest of your life.

Does the trainer personally write each program, or does he or she use generic one-fit-for-all?

There are websites on the Internet that trainers can use to create exercise routines for their clients. They can be very useful, with photographs and explanations for the exercises. No matter how good a routine is for one person though, it's not going to be suitable for every person. I write the program for a client's session each time individually, based on the results of the previous session.

A complete program can be produced based on the information from the consultation, but progress doesn't always proceed as planned. A good trainer will adjust the program session by session if necessary, to achieve optimum results.

Doe the trainer have the ability to clearly explain the exercise program?

A skilled trainer will be able to explain why a particular exercise is giving you a problem. He or she will then have the experience to know how to resolve it. A good trainer will always be happy to explain why it's important to do something a certain way. Your understanding of the mechanics of an exercise isn't necessary for you to perform it adequately. However, your understanding can go a long way to ensuring a safer and more effective exercise.

A good trainer will encourage feedback, and treat you with the utmost respect. Open communication between you and your personal trainer will result in a more rewarding experience for both of you.

Are your personal goals and limitations clearly defined during the consultation?

Everyone has a personal idea of what they want to achieve through an exercise program. More than likely there'll be more than one goal. I listed a few of them at the beginning of this segment. There'll be the long-term goal, such as reaching a particular weight or getting off of blood pressure medications. Then there'll be the short-term goal, such as fitting into a smaller outfit in time for a wedding.

Your trainer needs to help you set your goals realistically. Coaching you to achieve even more than you'd hoped for is the goal of a good trainer. Setting you up for disappointment is a waste of your time and money.

Does the trainer understand flexibility, and the important role that it plays in physical fitness?

I've worked alongside personal trainers who excelled in strength and endurance, but who had the flexibility of a steel bar! Muscle tension needs to be in balance if optimum strength, coordination, and power are to be achieved. A program that only focuses on strength, without considering muscle tension balance, can adversely affect your agility.

Understanding the importance of flexibility is also about stability and safety. This can improve your chances of avoiding injury. Stretching at the end of a routine has also been shown to help reduce the suffering of post-workout soreness.

Does the trainer focus on the client throughout the session without distractions?

I once watched a personal trainer reading the newspaper while her red faced, middle-aged client ran laps around the gym. If I were paying a trainer to work with me, I'd expect to have his or her undivided attention. Take the time to watch your prospective personal trainer working with current clients. Watch incognito if possible, so you can get a true picture.

During a session with a client, a good trainer will refrain from answering the telephone; reading the newspaper; drinking a cup of coffee; chatting to a friend walking by; or working on another client's program. You deserve the undivided attention of your personal coach; not only because you've paid for it - but for your safety!

SENSE AWARENESS

It's a lovely day, and three friends are sitting on the patio of a café having lunch together. The café sits on the corner of a huge intersection. Suddenly the pleasant afternoon is abruptly disrupted by a pickup truck running a red-light. The people sitting on the patio witness several cars piling up in the intersection directly ahead. If you were to ask the three friends what they observed, each one would describe the crash from a different perspective.

One of the three is more in-tune to sounds than to her other senses. She'll remember the banging and scraping noises over everything else. Her friend leans more towards smell-orientation; his olfactory sense is particularly keen. He may mention the strong smell of gasoline, as he recounts the event. The third member of the party is mostly sight-oriented. This friend will first recall the colors of the cars involved. Although being primarily sight-oriented is by far the most common, we're all a bit of a mixed bag when it comes to sense awareness.

A situation isn't actually something that you're involved in. A situation is something that you're creating through your subjective sensory experience. Working with a personal trainer, or working-out with a friend, is no different to any other situation in your life. You'll both be having a subjective experience of what you're doing together. That experience may not necessarily be in harmony.

Whether you're the client, the trainer, or the work-out buddy, it'll help you to understand how each person collects information uniquely. Working out together can be frustrating if you don't take individual sense orientation into consideration. A communication issue could be simply fixed by describing, as well as demonstrating an exercise to your client or partner.

You collect information through your six senses: seeing, hearing, smelling, tasting, touching, and intuiting. Smell, taste and intuition may seem unlikely to be exerting any influence when it comes to exercising, but don't underestimate the power that these senses have on your overall experience. It may be obvious that sight, hearing, and touch are required to perform your workout. But how you understand and retain information depends to some extent on all of your senses.

There are people who find it difficult to decipher written information. This can be a problem when sitting for an exam. In extreme cases the exam material has to be presented to them orally. This situation isn't a measure of their intelligence. It's simply a sign that he or she has an imbalance when it comes to sense awareness.

By practicing to improve one of your senses each and every day, you'll be able to reach a balance, or at least become closer to one. For example, to improve your hearing' orientation follow verbal directions only, without visual cues. The ultimate goal is to have all of your senses working at optimum efficiency, and in perfect harmony.

There are simple ways to tell which of your senses is primary. When putting together an 'assemble it yourself' piece of furniture, do you find it easy to follow the pictures and written instructions? If so, then you're more likely to be attuned to what you're seeing. There are people who can look at the pictures and read the instructions once, then build the item with ease.

Then there are people like me who have to read the instructions over and over again. I find it difficult to transfer what I'm reading to what I'm doing. Conversely, if someone reads the instructions out to me, I can follow the commands with no problem. Even as I'm writing this, I have to read it to myself out loud to determine if it conveys what I want to say.

If you struggle with pictures, written instructions, and also with verbal commands, then you may be 'feeling' dominant. Fortunately it's quite uncommon for the feeling sense to be the primary one. Education in our current culture revolves around books, computers, and television screens. These teaching aids are all primarily visual in nature, with auditory as a close second. Very little time, if any, is taken to nurture in a child the sense of 'feeling' his or her surroundings. This dominant reliance on vision is a major culprit in the balance and coordination issues that I come across in clients.

I had the challenge once of working with a client who was extremely feeling-oriented. Let's call her Joan. Joan came to me having held the belief all her life that she was stupid. She was uncoordinated, and had never mastered the simple act of catching a ball. Working together we found ways to improve her sight and hearing orientation. Playing a simple game of throw-and-catch with Joan was one of the most rewarding experiences of my career.

To improve your hearing sense orientation, record the following exercise. Then follow the verbal instructions. If you don't have a recording device, ask someone to read the instructions to you. You could also read them out loud to yourself.

ONE: Stand with your feet a shoulder width apart, toes facing forwards, and weight balanced between both feet.

TWO: Shift your weight to your left foot, and step your right foot straight back about two feet. Keep a shoulder width distance between the feet at all times.

THREE: Now balance your weight evenly between both feet again for the count of ten.

FOUR: Shift your weight back to the left foot, and step the right foot back to the original starting position.

FIVE: Stand with your feet a shoulder width apart, toes facing forwards, and weight balanced between both feet.

To improve sight orientation, perform the above exercise facing a mirror. Observe the position of your feet, hips, and shoulders at each point in the exercise. Notice if your feet are correctly pointing forwards. Are your shoulders and hips level? If not, then correct your position using your reflection in the mirror.

To improve feeling orientation, practice the exercise with your eyes open, then practice with your eyes closed. Shift your body weight back and forth between your feet, and notice how your body feels. Are you feeling pressure on the outside of your feet? Do your ankles fall inward? When practicing with your eyes closed pay particular attention to your posture. If closing your eyes makes you feel unstable, practice only with your eyes open. Have someone with you to ensure your safety. If necessary, place one hand on the wall.

If you enjoy group classes it's particularly beneficial to improve your overall sense orientation. An experienced teacher will not only give good visual demonstrations, but he or she will also provide excellent verbal directions as well. Not all instructors are experienced teachers though. Improving your sense orientation could be the difference between benefiting from a class, and dropping out of it altogether.

CREATING A WORKOUT ROUTINE

We live in a world of opposing forces, such as push and pull, raise and lower, back and forth. You can't enact opposing forces at the same time; in other words you can't push while you're pulling. The action of your muscles is no exception to this fact. For example, let's take flexing your biceps to bend your arm. The opposing muscles, the triceps, need to relax and stretch to allow your arm to bend.

There are many pairs of muscles, and groups of pairs, attached to each of your joints. It's not necessary for you to know the names and positions of each group. It's more important for you to know the correct range-of-motion of the joint. Too much flexibility can be just as detrimental as too little, as it can cause a joint to become unstable.

Exercising is a science. Certain things need to be understood if you intend to improve your strength, balance and flexibility. Working out without a basic understanding of what you're doing could easily cause more problems than it solves. If you're creating your own workout, ask yourself these questions before you begin any exercise in the routine:

How is this exercise going to help me with something that I do in my daily life?

Every week you are driving, gardening, shopping, vacuuming, changing cat litter, washing cars, moving furniture, and much more. These activities involve bending, twisting, squatting, pushing, and pulling. How is the exercise that you've added to your routine going to make these daily activities easier and safer for you?

Whether you run, golf, wrestle, dance, or sit on your butt all day, your activities could be messing with your muscular balance. Ask yourself if this particular exercise in the routine is going to help you to recreate balance, or just make a bad situation worse. You're in your body for the duration of your life. Taking care to balance those opposing forces now, can ensure that you still have your agility later on.

Can I do this exercise, with this particular weight, equally well on both sides?

Let's take for example that you choose a ten pound dumbbell to do a shoulder press. Watch yourself in the mirror as you perform the exercise. Both hands need to be in the same place at the end of the press. If one hand is higher than the other, you have an imbalance in muscle strength or flexibility. Notice if your shoulders are uneven, causing one hand to top out below the other, or perhaps one arm is bent at the elbow at a greater angle than the other.

Pay attention to the alignment of your trunk. Notice if you're leaning to one side as you press. If the answer is 'yes', then you have an imbalance in your trunk muscles that needs to be addressed. Only continue with this exercise if you can consciously fix a problem with ease while you're performing it. If you find yourself leaning backwards, turning the exercise into more of a chest press, lower the weight and try again.

Am I doing this exercise to create a healthy body, or just to create a certain look?

Men in particular will often work their chest, arms, and shoulder muscles, while neglecting their back, core, and legs. There's nothing wrong with wanting to look good, but it doesn't have to be at the expense of overall balance and fitness.

I was working in a gym when a bodybuilder asked me to help him with a problem. He was experiencing crippling lower back pain during his workout, and couldn't figure out why. I asked him to sit on a bench and demonstrate a shoulder press to me. He did so with ease, using fifty-pound dumbbells!

Next I asked him to show me a Plank Pose resting on his forearms. Plank is an effective core strengthening pose when performed correctly (without swayback). He was unable to even lift his hips up off the floor! After helping this young man with core strengthening and flexibility training, he was able to resume his body-building routine completely free of pain.

Am I doing this exercise just because it's easy, or because I don't know how to do anything else?

Creating a routine around what you find easy to do, is likely to exacerbate muscle tension imbalance. If you work out at a gym, look around you for people that are about your height, build, and fitness level. Pay attention to the exercises that they are doing. Also look for someone who's working with a trainer. Sit close by them for a while, and discretely observe. I reiterate here though that there's no substitute for working with a personal trainer yourself.

If you're creating your routine at home, then look up exercises on-line, or watch a TV exercise program. Always remember to use self-awareness when doing any exercise by yourself. You may look to be the same height, build, and fitness level as someone on the program, but you'll have your own unique challenges and limitations. And always remember, the instructor can't see you, so there's no one there to correct your form!

Am I doing this exercise to show off to someone else?

Working out with a friend can be a great incentive, or it can be your biggest problem. Western society is focused on competition, and I've witnessed people do crazy things because of it. When your attention is on showing off rather than on what you're doing, you're on a path to pain.

A yoga student will often look around her at other participants in the class. Then she'll push further into a pose in competition with a neighbor. The student will ignore the teacher affirming to stay at her own safe comfort level. The need to 'keep up with the pack' is a powerful incentive in a society that only rewards the winners. Anything less can create a feeling of failure.

For many people competition is all about respect. Do you really believe that if you can't leg press as much weight as your friend that you're not worth respecting? A more important question to ask yourself is what are you trying to achieve through exercising? When you rupture a disc because you're showing off to someone, you'll be losing a lot more than respect!

CORE MUSCLES

The word 'core' has become a buzzword in the exercise world today. Perhaps this is due to the emphasis placed on it by Pilates. I personally prefer the word 'trunk', as I think it's actually more accurate. For example: the core of an apple and the core of the Earth both imply that your 'core' is in the center of you. I've often been asked if back muscles are a part of the 'core'. No one's ever asked me if the back muscles are a part of the trunk.

I've encountered people who thought the core muscles were down the front of their abdomen. They believed that doing dozens of sit-ups and crunches every day was working their core. This is no different to believing that working only your biceps every day will strengthen and balance your arms. When you flex your abdominal muscles you're extending your back muscles, and vice versa.

If you were to Google 'core muscles' you'll find there is no defined list of which muscles actually belong to this group. Some sources believe that the buttocks are involved, some don't. Certain trainers include the mid-back muscles and thighs, some only the lower back. On one thing we all appear to agree though, muscles of your front, back, and sides are involved. To protect your spine and internal organs, all the muscles of your trunk, pelvis, and legs need to be exercised for optimum strength, flexibility, and safety.

If your workout consists of walking around the block, or playing tennis, is it necessary to have a strong core? The question needs to be in context to be relevant, because strength is relative. It isn't necessary to do sit-ups with a fifty-pound weight on your chest to play a good game of tennis. Come to think of it, it isn't necessary period! However, tennis calls for a variety of quickly changing jumping and twisting movements. Adequate strength and flexibility is required to protect your spine.

I recommend Hatha Yoga for working the muscles of the trunk. The body postures are designed to build strength and flexibility in balance, with the addition of body awareness. Hatha Yoga works the muscles in harmony; one group flexing and creating movement, the opposing group extending and allowing movement. The isometric contractions of certain poses also improve strength and stamina. This 'mindful' practice not only works the core to support the spine, it's designed to stabilize all of the joints of the body.

MACHINES VERSUS FREE-STYLE EXERCISE

Walk into any fitness club today and you're likely to be met by a row of weight machines called something like 'The Fast Line', or 'the Express Lane'. These machines are supposedly designed primarily for people who are: always in a hurry to be somewhere else; have marginal incentive to exercise at all; have plenty of time, but can't afford a trainer.

Ironically, despite their obvious appeal, machines are not ideal for beginners. You'll still need to know what you're doing to progress your workout safely. Machines don't call on you to work your core muscles for stability. The seating does that for you. Your core will become weaker in relationship to other muscle groups. This is exacerbated if an imbalance already exists. This kind of situation can put your back at risk for injury.

Another consideration is that there's no 'one-size-fits-all' machine. The seats and back supports will only move so high, or so low, and at the designated intervals. If the seat or back support isn't in the correct place for you, you'll develop an incorrect movement pattern to compensate. This kind of bad habit can be a 'fast track' to a chronic pain chain!

Weight machines are designed to work the major muscles of your body. The minor muscles that stabilize your joints and help you with balance are neglected. When working out with free-weights you have to stabilize yourself by using both minor and major muscle groups. If the allure of the easy machine line is just too great for you, then at least add a few core exercises as well. A well-conceived and varied routine can provide the necessary balance.

You'll still need to know what you're doing when you work out with free weights. At least you will if your goal is to have a safe and effective workout. I recommend a couple of sessions with an experienced trainer if at all possible. Ask the trainer why you're doing something a certain way, and what are the most important safety issues. Exercising with free weights ensures that you're working minor stabilizing muscles, as well as your major muscle groups.

If working with a trainer just isn't an option for you, then at least observe the following when you're using free weights:

1. Face a mirror so that you can watch what you're doing.
2. Whether you're sitting or standing, hold good posture at all times.
3. Breathe out as you exert yourself when working your chest or shoulders.
4. Learn from what others are doing around you, but don't compete with them.
5. If you're not sure how much weight to use, start with less and increase gradually.

Free weights aren't going to work directly the muscles of your hips, legs, and feet. Although you can work these particular muscles on fixed machines, lunges and squats can be a much better alternative. These multi-joint, multi-muscle movements will challenge your balance, and create strength with flexibility. Providing you're in a safe environment to do so, perform lunges and squats without shoes for added challenge. Exercising barefoot also strengthens and stretches the muscles of your feet and ankles.

Dr. Emily Splichal, a Podiatrist and Human Movement Specialist, teaches a certification course called, 'Barefoot Training Specialist'. Dr. Splitchal explains, "The foot has natural shock-absorbers that become weakened and less effective due to wearing shoes. Working out without footwear strengthens the muscles of the feet, and reactivates these shock-absorbers."

Of course, students have been practicing yoga barefoot for thousands of years!

FUN AND PLAYTIME

I'm seven years old and lying on my back on the village green. The only thought drifting through my mind is that of making shapes of the puffy clouds above. I'm sure that if you cast your mind back far enough, you'll find a similar memory tucked away in a drawer of your subconscious.

I'm not capable of being that clear minded today. Even though I practice yoga and meditation, the responsibilities of adult life still manage to worm their way into my thoughts. Besides, if the grown up me were to sprawl carefree on the village green today, a neighbor would call for the medics I'm sure!

Young children don't need to be taught how to relax, how to stretch, or how to exercise. It isn't necessary for them to use or understand the word 'exercise'. To a child, energetically exploring all that a body is capable of doing is called 'playing'. As that child matures into adulthood society teaches him how to behave in a more 'appropriate' manner. Propriety dictates that the free abandon of playtime is no longer appropriate.

The American Heart Association, and The American College of Sports Medicine, both recommend at least thirty minutes of moderate exercise per day to maintain good health. Medical research supports that a life devoid of exercise can lead to problems such as: Type II diabetes, heart disease, obesity, injury, and stress.

Another lifestyle related epidemic today is 'chronic pain'. Regardless of the cause, the results of chronic pain are the same as those of any other physical dis-ease: suffering, discomfort, and distraction. Chronic pain is often the result of a sedentary lifestyle. 'Exercise' has become such a dirty word to many people today that they'd rather suffer in silence, than find the motivation to be well again.

Because children don't think of exercising as a chore, they don't need motivating to take part in it. Outside my apartment window a group of young children are often playing under the trees. They jump up and down with long sticks, knocking the moss off the low hanging branches. I'm so tempted to grab a broomstick and gambol outside to join them. I don't do so of course, because it wouldn't be appropriate. God forbid should an adult jump around with such free abandon in public!

Why is it okay for a grown up to play something structured like softball, but not to play unstructured games like knocking moss off a tree branch? I'm not suggesting that you need to jump up and down with a stick to get your heart rate up. There's something to be said though for the children playing and laughing and having such fun. I'm sure that the word 'exercise' is nowhere to be found in their vocabulary. If your goal is to reclaim your fit and youthful self, then find something to do that's fun for you.

A mentor of mine once told me, "A person who exercises every day will never feel depressed." Over the years I've validated that statement for myself. Through regular and appropriate exercise I get better quality of sleep, and I feel agile, energized and relaxed. In my experience of working with clients, people who say to me, "I hate to exercise" are really saying one or more of the following:

I'm afraid of hurting myself.
I'm embarrassed because I sweat a lot.

I'm competitive, and I hate to appear weak.
I can't stop thinking about my responsibilities.
I'm uncomfortable with strangers looking at me.
I won't put my fat/skinny/ugly body in gym clothes.
I don't know what kind of exercise I should be doing.
I have way too much to do to waste my time exercising.
I was injured once, and don't want to go through that again.
I find walking boring, and don't know how to do anything else.

There was a time when poor posture and stiff joints were only afflictions of the elderly. Today such problems are affecting not only younger adults, but adolescents. Chronic pain is impacting people of all ages and social standing. Children are spending hours sitting hunched over some form or another of technology. Those children will progress into adulthood already burdened with chronic-pain-chains pulling them down.

When I first begin to work with a client, I rarely use any gym equipment. In fact, for some of the most important aspects of the training I use a tennis ball, a volley ball, and a piece of rope. With these simple tools I can coach my client to relax her mind using childhood games. A relaxed mind let's go of muscular tension. This in turn helps to improve balance, coordination, and agility.

As a pre-teen I spent hours bouncing a ball against the outside wall of the house. It was so much fun to hopscotch with nothing more than a piece of chalk. Can you imagine how a twelve year old would react today having nothing to play with but a piece of chalk? I'd bet she'd be complaining on social media before you could say 'click'!

Childhood itself seems to be an ever shrinking concept. Computer Science is frequently being taught in kindergarten; with Physical Education relegated to an optional status. Parents are ignoring their own need to exercise. How can they possibly motivate their children to do what they don't deem necessary for themselves?

A high percentage of children today are over-weight, and way too many are clinically obese. Making time every day for physical play is such a simple way to tackle these childhood problems. Yet it seems to be increasingly unthinkable in the minds of children, parents, and educators alike. For the sake of our society, if not for your own sake, don't just sit back and watch someone else play-ball!

DIET – IT'S A FOUR LETTER WORD

No book written about living blissfully in the body can be complete without a section on diet. After all, as the saying goes 'you are what you eat'. From my experience, how I fuel my body has a profound influence over how I feel. It amazes me that a doctor's office visit doesn't automatically begin with a diet questionnaire. In fact, I don't actually remember ever being asked about the foods that I consume!

I'm not a dietician, and I haven't come up with yet another fad diet to shed unwanted pounds. I haven't discovered an incredible way to lower my bad cholesterol, or overcome my diabetes. I can't talk heart to heart with you about our shared struggles with fluctuating weight either. This is because I've never actually experienced any of these problems.

What I can do is share with you how I've maintained a healthy weight for my height throughout my entire life. And my entire life now spans almost six decades. I can talk about why I've never been afflicted with a lifestyle related disease. Incidentally, my blood pressure has always been normal, and my back and knees are still doing just fine thank you!

Before I go any further, I'd like to make it clear that I'm not an alien from another planet. My genetics are as human as yours are. There's nothing different about the way that my body works. It's true that I can 'eat what I like' and still maintain a healthy body, because what I like to eat is healthy food. I can't eat food that's high in calories and low in nutrition, and not suffer the consequences, any more than you can.

The weight of your body, and the state of your body, are the result of what you think about. I've been talking about this from the beginning of the book, and there's nothing different going on here. Your diet is created by what you believe to be so, and what you decide to do with that information.

If you have a problem with your weight, high cholesterol, or Type II diabetes, take a candid look at what you're putting into your mouth. It's your mind that's creating your daily diet. Accepting this fact is the first step to gaining control over your wellbeing. The second step is taking a good hard look at what you're eating and why.

This may be the hardest part of the book for you to read. Food is closely tied into family, cultural, and social traditions and expectations. You might feel some unexpected emotions coming to the surface, such as indignation, guilt, or shame. There's no need to fight these feelings; learn about yourself from them instead.

All I can ask of you is that you read this entire section of the book to the end. Keep an open mind, and resist coming to any conclusions along the way. Let it sit with you for a day or two, and just observe the feelings that arise. Your daily diet can tell the story of your past, and in many ways it can predict your future!

YOUR WEIGHT IS NOT YOUR ENEMY

For as long as you live on this planet you're in your body; twenty four hours a day, seven days a week. How can you possibly live a life of bliss when every time you look in the mirror you see the enemy? The first step to achieving a healthy weight is to fully accept yourself: mind, body, and cellulite!

This concept is far from new of course. Self-help materials will teach you this at some point about any struggle in your life. Where you might trip up is in thinking that 'accepting' is the same thing as 'giving in', or even worse 'giving up'. On the contrary, accepting where you are right now is the only way to clearly see how you got there – and how to improve.

Accepting responsibility for every mouthful clears the way for you to consciously create your future diet. Taking a candid look at yourself will reveal your realization blind spots about your eating habits. The only 'good' diet is the one that supports your health and fitness for the rest of your life. To achieve this you'll need to be informed with reliable and ethical information.

Information that truly serves your health won't come from corporations with an interest in selling their products to you. TV commercials are there to boost the profits of the companies selling the goods. Don't be fooled into thinking that every claim they make must be true. Ad executives get paid big bucks to pull the wool over your eyes, and they've been doing it for years!

TEN EXCUSES FOR EATING AN UNHEALTHY DIET

The following are ten reasons that people have given to me for consciously choosing to eat an unhealthy diet. Have any of these excuses ever crossed your lips?

ONE: "I'M HISPANIC (ITALIAN, CHINESE, IRISH, SOUTHERN, ETC.) AND I WAS RAISED TO EAT THIS WAY."

My childhood meals included steak and kidney pie, fish and chips, and sandwiches made of a cow's tongue. There's no Universal Law that says I have to eat these meals today. I bet that wherever you're hanging your hat right now, you have access to the foods of many different cultures. I'd also bet that you're already incorporating their foods into your daily diet, and not always wisely.

In every corner of the world today you'll see the signs of fast food restaurants blighting the scenery. That doesn't mean that you have to eat at these places! Grocery stores everywhere now are selling a variety of produce from all over the world. Take advantage of the fresh fruits and vegetables available year round now. Who knows, you might even find a new favorite.

Two hundred years ago pilgrims were faced with hard winters, and little food to see them through to spring. They 'seasoned' their food with salt and fat to help preserve it, and to provide extra calories. They needed those calories to toil from dusk to dawn just to survive. There's no excuse today to 'season' your veggies with fat and salt, no matter where you were born. Unless of course you enjoy being overweight.

The Mediterranean peasant's diet of fresh greens and olive oil has morphed into heaps of pasta. Piles of spaghetti are topped with cream or tomato meat sauce, and smothered in cheese. This kind of meal is a veritable feast of simple carbs, saturated fat, and cholesterol! And pizza wasn't originally made with greasy cheese at all. Cheese was added by Americans in New York.

Even a light Chinese stir fry of seasonal vegetables has sunk into an oily mix of cheap meats. No matter which culture you were born into, times have changed. You have the chance now to choose the healthiest foods from an abundant worldwide bounty. You can still be healthy in today's society of quick, cheap, and nutritionally challenged. Base your diet on where you are right now; and toss your grandma's cookbook back in the attic.

TWO: "I CAN'T AFFORD TO BUY HEALTHY FOOD."

If you truly believe that you can't afford healthy food, then the problem is educational not financial. Foods that support a healthy body are: fruits, vegetables, beans, seeds, whole grains, and nuts. Foods that lead to obesity, low energy, and disease are: heavily processed foods; and those containing saturated fat, cholesterol, salt, white flour and sugar. But you already know this. So where did this idea come from that healthy foods are expensive?

Go back a few generations and you'll find a different approach to meal planning. Most families grew their own produce in backyard gardens. Processed food was minimal, and farms didn't have the word 'factory' in front of them. TV's and computers hadn't been invented yet, so vulnerable minds weren't being overwhelmed and tainted with misinformation.

As technology came along and whipped life into the fast lane, so did the need for faster meals. Along with this development came weight gain, health issues, and the onslaught of fad diets. Your grandparents didn't count calories, cut carbs, or pop pills to maintain a healthy body weight. That's not to say there weren't people who were overweight. Those that were though knew it was due to over indulgence, not ignorance.

Buying foods that support good health could save you a bundle in medical and pharmaceutical bills later on. To me this is reason enough to learn how to shop for healthy food on a budget. I'll do my best here to demystify the myths and misunderstandings rampant about food today. I'll site my sources when necessary, so that you can read the research for yourself. The pertinent question is, "can you afford not to eat well?"

Begin making changes gradually. Start by changing the ratio of foods on your plate. For example, if rice or pasta is a cheap staple for you, decrease the amount on your plate, and cook up frozen vegetables to mix in with it instead. Throw in a serving of kidney beans and you have a nutritionally complete and inexpensive meal.

Grocery stores are full of healthy, inexpensive foods if you take the time to look. You can even save money by eliminating things that you're simply eating out of habit. An example would be having bread with your pasta. Forget the bread, and buy only whole-grain pasta; it's more filling and more nutritious.

Put the money that you normally spend on bread towards fresh or frozen vegetables instead. Look for fresh fruits and veggies at local farmers markets, flea markets, and road side stands. Particularly if you go by them at the end of the day, they are practically giving their produce away.

Shop for fruits and vegetables that are in season at that particular time. Seasonal produce is fresh and abundant, and is going to be less expensive. For out of season produce check out the freezer section. I bought a bag of organic blackberries for $1.99 at a local supermarket the other day!

Many stores sell items in bulk bins; particularly 'health food' stores. You'll find rice, pasta, cereal, nuts, seeds, whole-grain flour, nutritional yeast, dried fruits, and much more. These foods will often be organic, unsulphured, and free of added sugar. Buying from bulk bins is less expensive than purchasing packaged foods.

There may not be many coupons available for healthy foods in the newspaper, but look for them in dispensers attached to the shelves at 'health food' stores. I've found coupons for a substantial amount off of the items being sold there. They also periodically have sales on organic frozen dinners. Stock up the freezer at this time.

Check out the 'health food' isle in your local grocery store. I've found whole grain, organic, and naturally sweetened products that are no more expensive than their unhealthy counterparts. Look for items on sale, and buy more than one.

This brings me to a point that I find most puzzling. Why would anyone shop in any other food isle than the 'health food' isle? I have to ask you "what's the alternative?" Perhaps if the meat section were labeled 'obesity and heart disease' it would be easier to avoid. If the dairy section had 'cancer and osteoporosis' overhead, you'd find it easier to pass on by!

There's no nutritional need to add chicken to a meal of beans and rice. A green vegetable is a much healthier choice. Vegetables are an important part of a balanced meal, not a 'side' to it. Top a grilled veggie burger with romaine lettuce, tomatoes, and avocado; a healthier and more delicious choice than fat, cholesterol, and calorie laden cheese.

THREE: "I DON'T HAVE TIME TO EAT FOODS THAT I KNOW ARE GOOD FOR ME."

If you believe that you don't have time to eat well, then again it's more an issue of education than it is of time. You develop your eating habits based somewhat on what you've learned from your family, friends, and peers. You're also influenced by commercials and other forms of media. The health of the populace has been steadily declining. It's now to the point where the importance of food choices can no longer be disregarded.

Commercials today are directing you more often to healthier choices in grocery stores and in restaurants. Even fast food establishments can no longer disregard the cries of an ailing nation. Drive-through burger joints are putting healthier choices on their menus in an effort to stay current. How much time do you need to choose a healthier item from the same menu?

Breakfast is the meal that usually goes by the wayside for time challenged people. Would you set out on a journey in your car without putting gas in the tank? Your metabolism will slow down and your energy level will drop if you don't eat regular meals. Breakfast can be something as simple as a banana and a handful of nuts; a piece of wholegrain bread and a tablespoon of peanut butter (no sugar or palm oil added); or instant unsweetened oatmeal with blueberries and almond milk.

Breakfast bars aren't something that I usually recommend, because most brands are little more than candy bars. Fruit and whole grains are a healthier way to start the day. Occasionally however, I'll resort to eating a bar in-between classes if I'm pressed for time. The only ones that I buy are made by 'Vega'. This brand offers a variety of different bars, shakes, and protein mixes. You'll find Vega products in health food stores.

Protein shakes are a popular way to start the day quickly for some people. I don't start the day with a protein mix myself; for me they are neither filling nor satisfying. If taking the time to eat a whole food breakfast is just out of the question for you, then Rainbow Light makes a good Protein Energizer shake mix. It's packed with nutrition provided by a variety of greens, as well as digestive enzymes.

Each bag of Rainbow Light Protein Energizer is stamped with the 'allergen safe guard', because this particular product contains plant based proteins. Rainbow stamps the 'allergen safe guard' on the Energizer mix because it doesn't contain whey. Whey is a by-product of processing cow's milk. Dairy products in general have been linked to food allergies. Pea and rice protein contains a complete amino-acid panel equal to whey.

Dairy protein has also been linked to cancer. 'The China Study', by Dr. T. Colin Campbell, is recognized as the most comprehensive study ever done on the relationship between diet and the risk of disease. During the study the following was discovered:

"Casein, which makes up 87% of cows milk protein, promoted all stages of the cancer process."

Why subject yourself to whey, an allergenic, and possibly carcinogenic milk by-product, when there's a healthier alternative?

There are days when I know that I won't have time to go home for lunch, or to stop by a restaurant that serves healthy food. So I take ten minutes in the morning to spread some hummus on two slices of Ezekiel bread, and top it with cucumber and tomato. Then I wrap it in cling-film and pop it into a small cooler. When lunch time comes around, every time I stop at a red light I take a couple of bites of my healthy sandwich. You couldn't get much more time-saving than that!

Hummus spread is available at just about every grocery store. You'll also find Ezekiel bread in the freezer (often in the vegetarian section) at most stores. It's more expensive than a loaf of bread from the isle, and about the same as a loaf of specialty bread at the deli. Ezekiel bread is made of sprouted grains and is free of flour, therefore it's low glycemic. This makes it more filling, and it won't have the effect on your blood sugar that bread made of flower has.

Flower bread usually also contains sugar or honey, particularly the wheat varieties. When you're used to the sweet taste of flower bread, it might take a bit of getting used to the change. Ezekiel has what I call a 'nutty' or 'grainy' texture. It reminds me of the fresh granary bread that I loved in England. Perhaps if you tried a slice with half a banana, or some other fruit, it might help you to make the transition.

Packing your own lunch is the best way of course to ensure a healthy meal. You don't have to take the time to make a sandwich. Keep some rice and peas aside from your dinner the night before; throw in some cashews and cilantro, and eat it cold for a balanced low calorie lunch. If you really don't want to take the time even for this, then buy a premade mixed salad or veggie sandwich from a deli or grocery store.

It takes discipline to change your eating habits. But first it takes the realization that you have the time to eat well if you really want to. It's nothing more than a habit when you place 'healthy eating' at the bottom of your priority list. Claiming that you don't have time to eat well is nothing less than a realization blind spot.

Trying to lose weight by not eating anything at all is equally unhealthy. Any weight that you manage to lose is likely to return. In the mean time you're starving your body of necessary nutrients. Eating small sized but calorie laden foods, such as burgers and milkshakes, is not the way to lose weight and keep it off either.

Eating five small, simple and balanced meals a day is a wise use of your time. You might want to think of it as three main meals and two smart snacks. A smart snack could be something like the following:

a) A banana with a slice of wholegrain bread (no butter) or a tablespoon of peanut butter
b) An apple with a handful of almonds or unsalted pumpkin seeds
c) Celery sticks dipped in garlic or red pepper hummus

Nurturing your body with as much live and whole food as possible will help you to achieve a healthy weight. Equally important, it will also create for you a healthy body in which to enjoy your life.

FOUR: "MY SPOUSE (ROOMMATE, PARENT, OR SIBLING) KEEPS UNHEALTHY FOOD IN THE HOUSE."

It goes without saying that you don't have to eat food just because it's there! So what's causing the real problem? Do you believe that healthy food is inferior in taste and smell to 'real' food? Does eating for health and wellness feel like a punishment that has to be endured? This kind of thinking can be programmed in to you over the span of your lifetime.

Notice how a commercial for cereal will make the statement, 'tastes so good even kids will eat it – but don't tell them that it's healthy too!' This statement implies that 'tasty' and 'healthy' are intrinsically opposed. Eating foods that are fatty, salty, or sweet can make it difficult to taste the subtle, yet delicious flavors of natural foods. It's your choice to hold on to the blind spot that whole foods are boring, tasteless or in some way less satisfying. Processed food producers are counting on you keeping that blind spot!

Choosing to remain ignorant allows you to blame someone else for your weight and wellness issues. If you're ready to break the programming, start buying your own foods today. Keep them next to the items that you've decided don't support your new healthy lifestyle. Perhaps you can inspire the people that you live with to break their programming too. There's no greater way to show your love for someone, than to inspire him or her to make healthier choices.

FIVE: "I DON'T EAT STUFF THAT'S BAD FOR ME; IT'S JUST THAT I EAT TOO MUCH."

An apple a day keeps the doctor away. This saying of course implies that apples are good for you. How many apples can you eat in one day? I'd imagine that you can't answer that question, because you've never tried to eat as many apples as you can in one day. Apples contain water soluble fiber that's great for your digestion. Eat too many apples at once however, and you'll be spending quality time in the bathroom!

What is it that determines if a particular food is 'good' or 'bad' for you? Well ask yourself this question, "does this food support the natural functions of my body, and if yes, how much of it do I need?" If you don't know how to answer the second part, imagine what it would be like if you ate nothing but that particular food all day long.

Brown rice is considered to be a healthy alternative to white rice. Does this mean then that a meal of five cups of brown rice is five times healthier than a meal of one cup? No it doesn't, because a healthy meal has a balance of fats, carbohydrates, and amino acids. A healthy meal also contains fiber, and a variety of essential vitamins and minerals.

Human beings are designed to eat a variety of foods, because all of our needs cannot be met by just one or two items. When you eat a sufficient variety to meet the needs of your body, you'll no longer be craving the things that it's possible to eat too much of.

Foods that support the natural functions of your body will be those that are rich in nutrients and low in calories. They'll also most likely be high in fiber and low in fat. Health forming foods will be vibrant and diverse in color; they'll leave you feeling satisfied without needing to feel 'full'.

Healthy foods will be fruits, vegetables, nuts, seeds, and whole grains, either uncooked or lightly cooked. Although raw foods have many benefits, cooked foods can be good for you in many ways too. Vegetables can be easier to digest when lightly stir fried, steamed, or stewed.

Dr. Joel Fuhrman, a medical doctor, nutritional researcher, and author of 'Eat to live,' and 'Nutritarian Handbook', has a 'raw verses cooked' page in the FAQ section of his website. He has this to say about the subject:

"Raw food is necessary for digestive efficiency, proper peristalsis and normal bowel function. Certain foods, especially fruit, avocado and nuts undergo significant change with cooking and are best eaten raw. Baking, frying, barbecuing and other high heat cooking methods that brown and damage food form acrylamide, which is potentially carcinogenic. Browning and other high heat cooking methods should be avoided. Cooking techniques like steaming vegetables, stewing foods in a pressure cooker and soup making, do not have these drawbacks. They do not brown foods or form acrylamide."

Nutritious food is minimally processed and will generally be free of white flour, sugar, dairy, saturated fat (with the exception of a small amount of coconut or avocado), and dietary cholesterol. If you're struggling with your weight because you're eating too much, I suggest that you re-evaluate the foods you're considering to be 'not bad for me'.

SIX: "I EAT UNHEALTHY FOOD, BUT I REALLY DON'T EAT THAT MUCH."

Deliberately depriving your body of good nutrition can be a form of self-abuse. Ask yourself this question, "when did I stop caring about myself?" Did it begin with an overly demanding job, or a family crisis? Did an unexpected change in your life make it difficult to eat as well as you did before? Try to figure out when and why you stopped making your health your priority. Only then will you know what to do to get back on track.

Then there are the diet plans on the market that actually tell you it's okay to eat unhealthy food, as long as you count the calories. They even sell packaged products that no one would ever mistake for healthy. It's okay to eat things like burgers and ice-cream cakes, as long as the calories are on the label. Stick to 'blah blah' number of calories a day, and you'll lose weight. What's your health got to do with it?

Let's not forget the carbs-cutting fads that have been around for a few decades now. The most well-known is probably the Atkins diet, first released in 1972. This particular diet approach is arguably the easiest to misunderstand, misuse, and deliberately abuse. I was sitting at a community kitchen table one day, when an extremely obese woman sat down beside me. I watched in confusion as she tossed away the bun, and proceeded to munch down on a double cheese burger.

"Atkins diet…" She announced with a grin. "I've lost three pounds this week!"

What she'd actually lost was three pounds of water from her cells. Consuming high amounts of protein can labor the kidneys. Not eating a variety of carbohydrates can also lead to insufficient vitamins, minerals, and fiber needed for a healthy body.

Your body turns carbohydrates into glucose, which provides your cells with the energy that you need to function. Not just energy for your skeletal muscles, but for your brain and nervous system as well. It's important however, to understand the difference between simple carbs, and complex carbs. When it comes to these low carb, high protein diets, it's also important to understand the construction of protein.

Simply carbohydrates are those that have been refined, such as white flour, white rice, and sugar. You'll find these products primarily in white bread, most crackers and cookies, pasta, cakes and puddings. No healthy, well balanced diet is going to place white bread and cake on the diet plan.

Fruit also contains simple carbs. The difference is that refined simple carbs have no fiber or nutritional value. For this reason they're considered 'empty calories.' Fruit on the other hand contains fiber, vitamins, and minerals, and is therefore a nutritious food. Fruit is best eaten in the morning, when you most need that boost of energy.

It isn't wise to consume a great deal of fruit, because it contains high calorie simple carbs. For this reason I don't advocate juicing, but prefer to make smoothies out of my fruit. A smoothie retains the fiber, and the vitamins and minerals that are found in the pith of the fruit too. Eating a piece of fruit as nature intended of course, is always the best option.

Complex carbohydrates are found in beans, peas, whole grains, and vegetables. As with fruits, these foods also provide fiber, vitamins, minerals and essential amino acids; the building blocks of protein. Breaking down the protein in meat and dairy takes a toll on your body. Animal products also contain saturated fats and dietary cholesterol, which can be detrimental to your health.

As I said before, you need carbohydrates to provide you with energy. You also need a small amount of fat to help with this process. When sufficient carbs aren't available, your body will turn to using protein and fat instead. Think of it as running out of wood for your fire. As an alternative, you throw an old tire on the embers. Yes, the rubber burns and produces some heat, but the purpose of rubber isn't to provide fuel. Eventually the toxic fumes will make you sick.

Even if you're not currently experiencing health or weight problems, give it time. Your body has an amazing ability to still function despite being poorly fuelled. The detrimental results may not be apparent at first, but inevitably they'll appear. Unfortunately, by the time you experience the deterioration of your cells, the damage will already have been done.

Eating heavily processed, fatty, or sugary foods, even in small amounts, causes your body to become acidic. Acidity can lead to osteoporosis, arthritis, infection, and many other health related problems. Only you can decide to make better dietary choices for yourself. Don't wait for your apathy to turn into regret.

SEVEN: "I HATE COOKING."

If you eat out in restaurants - you can eat healthy in restaurants! Every item found in every dish on the menu is being prepped in the kitchen. All it takes is a little creativity. Ask for roasted vegetables on top of rice and beans. Ask for a stir-fry of all of the vegetables on the menu, and add mushrooms. Tell the server that you'd like a meal that doesn't contain white flour, saturated fat or cholesterol. I've never yet come across a chef that isn't happy to help me with my requests.

While you're out for dinner, ask for beans and rice or a vegetable stir-fry to go. Now you have lunch ready for the next day. Grocery stores and delis sell premade sandwiches and a variety of salads ready to go. Fruit doesn't need to be cooked. Complete inexpensive meals can be purchased in Café's, smoothie bars, and health food stores in just about every town.

Buy dried fruit, nuts, and seeds (no sugar or salt added) from the bulk bins, and make your own trail mix. Eat instant unsweetened oatmeal (just add boiling water) for breakfast with juicy fresh berries, or a banana. Make peanut butter (no added sugar or palm oil) and banana sandwiches on whole grain bread. Note that 'whole wheat' bread is not the same as 'whole grain'. Some whole wheat breads are nothing more than white bread with brown coloring.

If money is a concern, choose frozen dinners and packaged soups. There's no need to skip on quality here either. I enjoy Dr. McDougall's soup in a box, found at health food stores. My favorites are black beans with rice, minestrone, and lentil. I add a couple of slices of Ezekiel bread. The only frozen dinners that I buy are Amy's brand. The food inside the box actually looks the way it does on the front cover. I've found this to be unusual with frozen dinners. Amy's are organic to boot.

Amy's frozen dinners and soup cans are sold not only in health food stores, but at most major grocery stores too. You can sometimes find Dr. McDougall's products in general grocery stores, but will usually find them in health food stores. Dr. McDougall also has a great website packed with products and nutritional information: www.drmcdougall.com.

Finding no pleasure in the culinary arts doesn't give you a free pass to make unhealthy choices. Use your imagination, be creative, or just make a better effort. It doesn't take a chef to heat up some frozen veggies, boil a serving of brown rice or quinoa pasta, and sprinkle some nutritional yeast on top. If you prefer a sauce over your pasta and veggies, mix the nutritional yeast with a little water for a 'cheesy' tasting topping. You could also just use a traditional tomato sauce.

Nutritional yeast can be found in health food store bulk bins, where it will be less expensive than buying it prepackaged. I regularly sprinkle these tasty golden flakes on my salads, as well as over my vegetables and quinoa pasta. Quinoa is actually a seed, not a grain, therefore it's gluten free and high in protein. You can find Quinoa products at most grocery stores in the 'gluten free' isle.

Having no incentive to cook can lead to a healthier diet than if you were a master chef. Fruits, salads, nuts, and seeds need no cooking, and provide you with nutrients and fiber. Frozen vegetables and pasta made of brown rice or ancient grains take just ten minutes in boiling water. Throw in canned beans and you have a nutritionally complete, filling, and low fat meal. It takes no more time and effort than ruining your health at the fast food drive though!

EIGHT: "I DON'T KNOW HOW TO EAT ANY OTHER WAY."

The likelihood of this statement actually being true is minimal. It's probably more accurate to say, "I'm a bit scared of how I'm going to feel if I change what I'm eating." Regardless of how poor your diet may be, sticking with 'the devil you know' can be less intimidating that trying something different.

There could be good reason for this concern too if you're currently living on stodgy, high fat foods. Suddenly adding fiber to your daily diet could lead to some embarrassing moments. It's wise to make the changes to your diet gradually.

If your breakfast usually consists of doughnuts, then switch to sweetened apple and cinnamon oatmeal instead. After a week, start mixing three quarters of the apple and cinnamon with a quarter of plain oatmeal together. One more week later mix half and half of the two types of oatmeal together. You get the picture.

When it comes to making a salad, the darker green the lettuce the more nutritious it is for you. Iceberg lettuce is the least expensive, and therefore usually the most popular. Unfortunately, it's the least healthy choice for you to make too. Romaine is the highest in vitamins and fiber; with butterhead lettuce not far behind.

Top your salad with lightly steamed cut green beans instead of sweet corn. Sweet corn is difficult to digest, and has a lower nutritional value than green beans. I enjoy the heads of asparagus on my salad, along with avocado, tomato, and cucumber.

Slices of raw or lightly steamed beets add a deep red to the mix, along with iron and a variety of other vitamins and nutrients. Mix as many colors as you can for your salad, and you'll be treating yourself to all of the amino acids required to make protein.

Adding butter or bacon to vegetables may be a common practice in your family. If so, cut down gradually on the amount that you're adding. In time you'll be surprised at just how delicious vegetables taste without saturated fat slathered all over them. You may even discover a new love in your life!

You may experience discomfort at first when you start adding more fiber to your diet. This is by far outweighed by the many advantages for your health. Foods that contain fiber also contain the nutrients that your body needs to maintain good health and wellness.

Cut down on sugar, saturated fat, and salt in your diet, and increase the fresh fruits, whole grains, and vegetables. By making this simple shift you'll soon notice an increase in your energy level. Depending on just how poor your diet was to begin with, you may also notice improvements in your skin, hair, and nails.

What you see on the surface of your body is a reflection of what's happening inside you as well. Changing your diet is going to take desire and motivation, as well as information. If for no better reason, don't you want to look and feel better? If so, stop using ignorance as an excuse to choose an unhealthy diet. Start using self-preservation as an inspiration to change your life.

NINE: "I'M AN EMOTIONAL EATER, AND I LOVE SWEET [FATTY OR SALTY] FOODS."

This claim is propagated and validated by the writers of TV programs and movies. Two or more women, and for some reason it's usually women, sit down to a pity party with a gallon of ice-cream. Watching a scene like this reinforces your belief that emotional eating is normal behavior. Well, it may be a normal way for some people to react, but it's far from natural.

When you're emotionally upset, your body experiences physical stress. The last thing you need at this time is to stress your body even further with fat and sugar. A lifelong habitual response can be tough to shake though; it's going to take some training on your part.

The term 'comfort food' means different things to different people. If you're having weight or health problems because you consider yourself to be an emotional eater, try writing the words 'comfort food' and then 'healthy food' on two different pieces of paper. Under the heading on each page, write what each of those words currently mean to you.

The positive thing about the statement "I'm an emotional eater" is that you're aware of what you're doing. The negative aspect is not realizing that this behavior is nothing more than a realization blind spot.

Your emotions result from what you think and choose to believe. When you believe that you need a certain food to make you feel better, you'll always find an excuse to indulge yourself with that food. To begin creating a healthier habit around your emotions, stop buying whatever you consider your 'comfort food' to be. This will be the first step, and the first challenge to overcome.

Next time you reach for that gallon of sweet frozen appeasement ask yourself these questions: "What do I really want to feel? Will eating this heal my relationship? Will it put money in my purse? Will eating this unhealthy food fix any of the challenges in my life right now? Can I accept that eating this won't ease my pain, but will only make me feel worse by causing fatigue and weight problems?"

If you want things in your life to change, then change things in your life. Start with what you're buying to stock your pantry. A grocery list of healthy choices doesn't have to be devoid of foods that you love. You will however need to question yourself as to why you love that particular food.

There are times when people habitually eat junk food as a social expectation. For example, do you eat a bag of popcorn at the movies? Is it the norm for you to grab a hotdog at the ballgame? Are there restaurants known for their pies, so you just have to have a piece when you go there? Have you ever even asked yourself why you 'love' eating this unhealthy food?

Saying 'no' to a piece of cake, a cheese burger, or a bag of chips can actually feel distressing for some people. If this is you, then the issue may be more involved than it appears to be on the surface. Your subconscious mind is incredibly strong. To make you feel better when you're feeling stress, your subconscious may recall birthday parties, family fun days, and celebrations.

In western society joyful celebrations revolve around the unhealthiest foods available. Perhaps next time you find yourself drawn to something sweet, fatty, or salty because you 'love' it, pause before you put it in your mouth. Allow yourself to truly feel what comes up when you resist.

It may appear to you that you've no control over the foods you love to eat. Truthfully, you can easily change taste preferences by changing the foods in your refrigerator. I used to absolutely love Cheddar cheese and milk chocolate. Then I found out that dairy was causing my debilitating migraines.

Having been totally off of dairy now for many years, the very thought of greasy cheese makes me nauseated. It's hard for me to believe now that I ever 'loved' the taste of this product. Thankfully, I can still eat dairy free chocolate without a problem -there is a God!

If I can improve my life by changing my diet, then you can too. If you're an adult, only you are controlling what goes into your mouth. Decide to eat consciously, and discover a whole new world of nutritious foods to fall in love with.

TEN: "I'D LIKE TO EAT A HEALTHY PLANT BASED DIET, BUT I'M CONCERNED ABOUT NOT GETTING ENOUGH PROTEIN."

I doubt that your great grandparents gave any thought to how much protein they were eating each day. I also doubt they could tell if they were getting the correct percentage of DV (daily value) of vitamins and minerals either.

Traveling between time zones was more difficult when your great grandparents were youngsters. People in general ate seasonal and locally grown produce. Meat was usually the most expensive part of the meal, and therefore the smallest.

With the advent of factory farms, refrigerated trucks, and fast food restaurants, the balance of the average meal has changed. It takes time and money to cut up fruits and vegetables, and to bake whole grain breads and pasta. Fast food restaurants save money by using the cheapest ingredients they can buy. They serve food that is quick to prepare, and easy to eat on the go.

The problem of poorly balanced nutrition is aggravated by government subsidizing of the meat and dairy industries. The chart on the website for PCRM (Physician's Committee for Responsible Medicine) shows that sixty three percent of subsidies go to the meat and dairy industry, while only one percent goes to fruits and vegetables.

It's commendable that many physicians now recognize the role of diet in the most common chronic diseases. Yet physicians in the west receive little, if any training in diet and nutrition. What they do know is often out of date, and commonly out of context. This little bit of knowledge can be a dangerous thing, when it's being taught to trusting patients.

Commercials for food on TV are paid for by companies promoting their products. The information being presented is accepted by viewers as fact. Whereas the fact is that the information is frequently misleading, and often down right wrong. Add to this the fad diets that come and go, and the 'Protein Myth' is propagated.

It's true that meat and dairy products contain all nine essential amino acids required to make protein. However, not all amino acids required to make protein are contained in meat and dairy. This is the first part of the myth. The second part of the myth is that the human body needs huge amounts of protein to be healthy.

More animal protein is consumed in the US today than anywhere else on the planet. Animal products also contain saturated fat and cholesterol. Unfortunately, the rest of the globe is fast catching up with this heavy consumption. Most people are eating far more protein than their body needs, or can safely digest and dispose of.

This is taken from the American Heart Association article, HIGH PROTEIN DIETS, January 3rd, 2012:

"These [high protein] diets can cause a quick drop in weight because eliminating carbohydrates causes a loss of body fluids. Lowering carbohydrate intake also prevents the body from completely burning fat. In the diets that are also high in protein, substances called ketones are formed and released into the bloodstream, a condition called ketosis. It makes dieting easier because it lowers appetite and may cause nausea.

Most Americans already eat more protein than their bodies need. And eating too much protein can increase health risks. High-protein animal foods are usually also high in saturated fat. Eating large amounts of high-fat foods for a sustained period raises the risk of coronary heart disease, diabetes, stroke and several types of cancer. People who can't use excess protein effectively may be at higher risk of kidney and liver disorders, and osteoporosis."

Proteins are actually made up of various combinations of twenty nine amino acids. Your body makes twenty of them itself. Only the other nine need to be consumed in your diet; these are called the 'essential amino acids'. Plant foods all contain one or more of the essential amino acids. Eating a variety of colors and textures in your daily diet ensures that your body is receiving sufficient protein.

At one time it was thought that if you work-out you need to eat much more protein than when you're sedentary. Two decades ago it wasn't unusual for athletes and body builders to gorge on 'steak and eggs' for breakfast. Current research into health and fitness no longer supports that this is necessary.

Increased activity calls for eating more of everything that your body needs to maintain good health. Maintaining the correct balance of carbohydrates, protein, and fat is the key. Research supports that consuming large amounts of animal protein is detrimental for everyone, regardless of their level of fitness. Animal products also contain unhealthy saturated fat, and are the only source of dietary cholesterol. Not to mention the added antibiotics, steroids, and hormones.

Your body needs carbohydrates to produce energy. Protein is used to repair tissue. Weight lifting causes your muscles to 'get bigger' through hypertrophy. What's actually happening is that you're tearing the fibers of your muscles. Those tears are then repaired with protein, forming scar tissue which builds bulk.

There are some incredible athletes and competition body builders enjoying a plant based diet. They aren't just maintaining a healthy nutritional balance; they're thriving in the athletic arena. The following are just a few of these people:

EMILY JANS: National Boxing Champion
CARL LEWIS: Winner of nine Olympic Gold Medals
KENNETH G. WILLIAMS: American Bodybuilding Champion
MAC DANZIG: Internationally recognized Mixed Martial Artist
BRENDAN BRAZIER: World Champion Triathlete and Endurance Runner
PATRIK BABOUMIAN: Germany's Strongest Man, and World Record Holder for Log Lift

Perhaps you're still not sure that protein isn't really what you thought it was. Your still not convinced that you don't need eggs, meat, or dairy at every meal. Changing a life-long habit can be a tall order; even if that habit has the potential to cause a lifestyle related disease.

From where do you think other animals get their protein? Not carnivores like tigers and lions; I'm talking about herbivore animals. How do they manage to get enough protein? There are some incredible non-human athletes and body builders thriving on a plant based diet. Every one of them consumes plenty of protein to maintain a huge and healthy body:

ELEPHANT: Strength and Endurance. An elephant, the largest land mammal, not only has the strength to knock down a tree, but can pick up over six hundred and fifty pounds with his trunk.

GORILLA: Strength and Agility. A gorilla has six times the upper body strength of a human male, while still being able to move with graceful ease.

RHINOCEROS: Power and Speed. A rhinoceros can range in weight from fifteen hundred pounds to three tons, and can charge at speeds of up to forty-five miles per hour.

PRONGHORN ANTELOPE: Speed and Endurance. A pronghorn antelope can run up to forty miles per hour for over four miles without stopping.

GIRAFFE: Kick Fighter. A giraffe has a power kick that can decapitate a lion.

HORSE: Sprinter. Horses can run between thirty and fifty miles per hour over short distances.

CAMEL: Endurance Runner. A camel has been recorded covering a distance of six miles in less than twenty minutes. They can also walk for days in temperatures over 100F without water.

COW: Track and Field: A Cow can jump a six foot fence, and trot for miles.

As you can see, some of the largest, strongest, and fastest animals in the world are getting their protein totally from plant foods. You too can adopt a healthier, low fat and cholesterol free diet without worrying about getting enough protein. All you have to do is eat a wide variety of live and minimally processed foods.

Plant sources that contain the highest number of amino acids are: beans, peanuts, lentils, soybeans, tofu, tempeh, and nuts. However, fruits, grains and vegetables also contain a significant variety. By increasing the amount that you eat of all of the above, you'll increase your overall protein intake. In addition, you'll be increasing all of the other essential nutrients that your body needs for wellness.

A well-rounded diet negates the necessity to add protein powder to your meals. This is particularly true of whey powder, a by-product of processed milk. The extensive research done in the 'China Study' linked the proteins in milk to 'turning on' cancer cells.

PCRM (Physicians Committee for Responsible Medicine) created a list of the health risks associated with eating too much dietary protein: kidney disease, kidney stones, osteoporosis, and cancer. The following is a quote from the nutrition experts at PCRM:

"To consume a diet that contains enough, but not too much protein, simply replace animal products with grains, vegetables, legumes (peas, beans, and lentils), and fruits. As long as one is eating a variety of plant foods in sufficient quantity to maintain one's weight, the body gets plenty of protein."

FIFTEEN REASONS FOR CHOOSING A HEALTHIER DIET

We've just explored the excuses that people make to eat what they know isn't good for them. Now let's take a comprehensive look at fifteen reasons to eat healthier from now on.

ONE: YOU WANT TO AVOID GETTING A LIFESTYLE RELATED DISEASE, SUCH AS TYPE II DIABETES, HEART DISEASE, OR OBESITY.

It's no big secret, or a surprise that as the quality of food goes down, the number of lifestyle related diseases goes up. The problem is multifaceted. There are the many forms of sugar for example, including corn syrup and molasses. Also high up on the list of poor quality foods you'll find: saturated fat, trans fat, and GMO (genetically modified organisms).

One might believe that fear of disease would be incentive enough to make healthier choices. The rising number of lifestyle related epidemics would indicate the contrary. Perhaps this is because of an even more common affliction, the one known as 'it won't happen to me' syndrome.

You don't develop heart disease after eating one meal. You don't catch Type II Diabetes from a grocery store shopping cart. What you put into that cart for dinner however, is a very different story. The AHA (American Heart

Association) and the ADA (American Diabetes Association) both recognize the importance of dietary choices.

Both the AHA and the ADA recommend a diet rich in fruits, vegetables, nuts, seeds, and whole grains. Yes, even the American Diabetes Association recommends twenty-eight fruits on its list of healthy foods! The following is from the ADA website for people who are already suffering from diabetes:

"Wondering if you can eat fruit? Yes! Fruits are loaded with vitamins, minerals and fiber just like vegetables. Fruit contains carbohydrate so you need to count it as part of your meal plan. Having a piece of fresh fruit or fruit salad for dessert is a great way to satisfy your sweet tooth and get the extra nutrition you're looking for."

In this case, like never before has an ounce of prevention been worth a pound of cure. When it comes to avoiding a major lifestyle related disease, an ounce of healthy food is worth a pound of pharmaceutical medications!

TWO: YOU HAVE A LIFESTYLE RELATED DISEASE, AND YOUR DOCTOR HAS TOLD YOU TO LOSE WEIGHT.

When it comes to losing weight, the bottom line is that you need to be using more calories than you're consuming. You won't lose weight by skipping meals altogether though; even though it may sound good in theory. Initially you may experience a little weight loss. But if you continue to deprive your body of food, it will respond by lowering your energy level. You'll achieve nothing more in the long run than chronic fatigue.

There've been more fad diets on the market than there are cookie recipes! Some of them attempt to hook you by declaring that "it isn't your fault that you're overweight." It's not about fault, but it is about responsibility. How can your body weight be the result of anything other than your lifestyle and dietary choices? A fad diet isn't going to create a healthy body for you because you've found something else to 'blame'.

There are some medical conditions that can lead to weight gain, but they're relatively rare. Your physician can easily rule them out, along with any medications that could be responsible. Stress can lead to over-eating and over production of the hormone cortisol. Cortisol is believed to be responsible for storing excess belly fat. Relieve the stress in your life by adding yoga and meditation to your daily routine.

Learn from what you've done in the past. If your doctor is recommending that you lose weight, it's time to make better lifestyle choices. Choose foods that are high in nutrition, high in fiber, and low in calories. Healthy foods are the ones as close to being whole and alive as possible: fruits, vegetables, nuts, seeds, and grains.

Foods to avoid are those that are highly processed, high in calories, and low in nutrition and fiber. Such items will contain refined sugar, corn syrup, white flour, hydrogenated and saturated fats, and dietary cholesterol.

The knowledge that you already have is your most useful tool. A friend of mine claimed that she had no idea why her body weighed almost four hundred pounds. Perhaps she didn't know that eating enough pasta at one meal to feed ten people would cause weight gain. I'd bet the bank though that she knew the ice-cream for dessert was loaded with empty calories.

When you choose foods that are nutritious, filled with fiber, and low in calories you can eat more food more often. Three to five small balanced meals per day are preferred over one large meal. Your body will have all that it needs for optimal function, so your metabolism will become more efficient. The result is that your vitality goes up, and your weight goes down!

THREE: YOU'RE OVERWEIGHT, AND IT'S CAUSING
PROBLEMS WITH YOUR KNEES.

Your knees are vulnerable joints no matter how much
you weigh. The fittest athletes can injure their knees playing
physically active sports. Knee pain is often chronic though,
and not related to an injury. This type of pain chain is often
the result of tight and weak hip muscles. Weak and tight
muscles of the calves and ankles can also be involved. No
matter what the cause of the pain, being overweight is only
going to exacerbate the problem.

Start by cutting calorie dense fatty and processed
foods out of your diet, and adding more live fruits and
vegetables. Making this simple lifestyle change has more than
one advantage. Not only will you drop those extra pounds,
you'll be improving the health of your bones, ligaments, and
tendons. If your joints themselves are unhealthy, achieving
that ideal weight isn't going to be much of an advantage.
Eating a variety of plants provides the nutrients that your cells
need for maintaining healthy joints.

The majority of people know of course that calcium is
a necessary mineral for your bones. What they often don't
know is that your body also uses calcium to balance the pH of
your blood. Research now confirms that consuming calcium
via dairy products isn't the wisest choice to make. Dairy
causes your body to become acidic. Acidity pulls the calcium
right out of your bones, and into your blood stream to balance
the pH.

Dark leafy greens are high in calcium, which your
body can easily utilize. Dark greens are also alkaline, and
therefore won't interfere with the pH balance of your blood.
Dairy contains cholesterol and fat (even the low fat variety).
And unless you're buying organic every single time, you're
consuming hormones that are playing havoc in your body.
Vegetables are low in calories, free of fat and hormones, and
packed with a variety of nutrients and fiber.

How I've kept a healthy weight my entire adult life is
no great secret. I love dark leafy greens, cooked with just a

pinch of unrefined salt (I use Redmond sea salt), and a teaspoon of apple cider vinegar. The vinegar cuts the bitterness and brings out the natural delicious flavor of the greens. Apple cider vinegar has also been frequently reported to help with arthritis.

When you plan a meal think about how you can eliminate, or at least lower, the highest calorie component of it. There's no need to add the empty calories of a piece of fatty pork hock to your leafy greens. Then look at increasing the foods with the highest nutritional value. Your knee bones will thank you for it!

FOUR: YOU WANT TO LOOK AND FEEL BETTER IN YOUR CLOTHES – AND OUT OF THEM!

Your self-image is a creation of your mind. In other words it's your own opinion of what your body currently looks like. Your body is the result of your lifestyle. How you see it will depend on several factors, including the influence of your family and friends, and the society in which you live. What you do about it is entirely up to you. If looking in the mirror leaves you feeling dissatisfied, think of yourself as standing at a fork in the road.

The left-hand fork leads to a place called 'Self-Pity'. Self-pity is a heavily populated area, so at least you'll always have company! Once there you'll find plenty of ways to indulge yourself, perpetuating your judgment of poor self-image. The problem with this destination is that although it's easy to arrive at, it's very difficult to find your way out again.

The right-hand fork leads to 'Determination'. When you chose Determination, you'll find it comes with a map marked, "you are here". Starting from the point marked clearly on the map, the road to follow becomes surprisingly clear. Determination is a place where you find healthy meals, walking paths, and encouraging affirmations. The longer you stay in Determination, the more improvement you get to see in your reflection!

FIVE: YOU WANT TO IMPROVE YOUR SKIN TONE, AND AVOID AGE SPOTS (ALSO KNOWN AS LIVER OR SUN SPOTS).

Your skin is the largest organ of your body. It's akin to a sponge, soaking up everything that you rub, spread, and spray on it. What you're feeding your skin from the inside is of equal importance to what you put on the outside. This vital organ is made up of trillions of cells. To protect these cells from being damaged by free radicals and the radiation in sunlight, you need to provide it with antioxidants.

Dark leafy greens such as kale, cabbage, and spinach all contain antioxidants. A variety of fruits are rich in Vitamin C. This crucial vitamin is not only an antioxidant, but also necessary for building the collagen that gives your skin its elasticity. Collagen strengthens the capillaries that fill with blood to feed the nutrients to your skin.

Orange colored vegetables such as carrots and cantaloupe not only contain vitamin C, but are also high in beta carotene. Your body converts beta carotene into Vitamin A, a necessary nutrient to repair and maintain healthy skin. A variety of grains such as barley and millet contain not only vitamins, but the minerals necessary for the healthy production of your cells.

Don't underestimate the power of nuts either when it comes to a healthy skin. You may already be aware of the benefits of almonds, cashews, and walnuts. Often overlooked though are Brazil nuts and macadamias, both of which are touted for being excellent for your skin. Nuts also contain monounsaturated and polyunsaturated fats; the 'good' fats that your body needs to maintain a healthy state.

Avocado is another excellent source of the 'good fats'. Often referred to as a 'super-food', avocado provides about twenty vitamins and minerals, such as lutein, a nutrient that's excellent for your eyes. Recipes for making your own face mask often include avocado. The nutrients can be absorbed through your skin from the outside, in addition to being ingested.

Your skin is exposed to toxins just by living in the world today. You can help yourself though by avoiding items that contain preservatives, colors, or synthetic perfumes. Even a product that claims to be 'all natural', or to be 'aromatherapy' contains chemicals if you also see the word 'perfume'. Products containing perfume make me sneeze; on the other hand, true essential oils don't bother me at all.

An excellent way to introduce nutrients to your skin is through Abhyanga. Abhyanga is a form of nurturing self-massage practiced in Ayurveda, the ancient healing science of India. The traditional oil to use with an Abhyanga massage is sesame oil, which can be infused with essential oils if desired. Sesame oil is considered to be one of the most powerful antioxidants available. The benefits of sesame, according to Ayurveda, are even more effective when applied topically than when consumed.

You'll need organic, cold pressed sesame oil for Abhyanga practice. This oil is golden in color; unlike the dark brown toasted sesame oil used in cooking. If you're allergic to sesame, you can use an alternative massage oil in its place. Ask at your local health food store for help in choosing the right oil for you. The massage will be just as effective.

Here are directions for performing Abhyanga self-massage:

STEP ONE: Warm the oil for the massage; you'll only need a couple of ounces. You can place the glass container in some hot water to warm the oil. I like to rub some between my hands to warm it up.

STEP TWO: Gently rub the oil into your skin; using less is better than more. On the straight parts such as arms and legs, rub the oil vigorously in straight lines. On the joints of your body such as elbows and knees, rub in circular clock-wise motions.

It's okay to have someone help you with the difficult to reach areas of your body. If no one is available to help you, just massage the areas that you can reach by yourself. Massage a little oil into your scalp for an excellent hair tonic!

STEP THREE: Allow the oil to soak into your skin for at least ten minutes. Then take a warm shower or bath. If you don't mind the feeling of the oil on your skin, you can leave it on for as long as you like.

This healing and self-nurturing practice not only feeds your body with antioxidants, it leaves your skin feeling soft and youthful.

Being of Northern European descent, my skin has a tendency to be dry. Whether your skin is dry or not though, keeping it hydrated is equally important for everybody. If you don't care to drink clean fresh water, at least avoid caffeinated drinks. Caffeine is a diuretic which is counterproductive to hydrating your skin. Eat juicy fruits and vegetables that naturally contain water, and drink green or herbal teas. I don't advise drinking fruit juice, as it contains too high a concentration of sugar.

Liver spots, also known as age or sun spots, appear to be a bit of a mystery. According to the Mayo clinic they have nothing to do with the liver at all. Sun spots, as they refer to them, may be due to hereditary factors and sun exposure. However, they don't know for sure what causes this phenomenon. Another medical explanation is that these grey, black, or brown spots may be due to toxic buildup in the liver over time. The toxic buildup theory could explain why 'age spots' tend to appear on people over forty years of age.

Most medical sources agree that sun exposure is the trigger, if not the cause. This is because liver spots are customarily found on the back of the hands and on the face. These areas are most likely to be exposed for long periods of time to the ultraviolet rays of the sun. The good news is that although liver spots may be unsightly, they're quite harmless. The bad news is that the only way to get rid of them is with some kind of bleaching agent.

Whether you call them liver, age, or sun spots, if they appear I suggest that you show them to your physician. These skin anomalies could be masking skin cancer, such as melanoma. Melanoma is a serious problem that can be successfully treated if caught early on.

The health of your skin is a reflection of the health of your organs in general. Youthful and protected skin is one that's hydrated, nurtured, and nutritionally supported. By taking good care of your skin, you'll be improving your overall health and wellbeing.

SIX: YOU WANT TO EXERCISE MORE, BUT YOU GET OUT OF BREATH EASILY.

Although it should go without saying, I'll say it anyway; consult with your physician if you're getting out of breath. There are many conditions that can challenge your breathing when you increase your activity level. One such condition is exercise-induced asthma; another is an allergic response.

You could be allergic to something that you're eating. Allergies and sensitivity to food can also lead to inflammation and weight gain. A true food allergy causes your body to respond in the way that it does to any allergy; there'll be symptoms such as: hives, itchiness, breathing difficulties, sneezing and coughing. Allergies can be serious business, and can worsen quickly.

Food sensitivity can be similar to an allergic response, but it isn't the same. The symptoms can include: bloating, stomach cramps, and diarrhea. If you're in any doubt as to whether you're sensitive to something in your diet, or whether you have an allergy to a food, get yourself tested by a professional. The following are just some of the foods commonly associated with sensitivities and allergies:

Dairy (includes milk, cheese, ice-cream, yogurt and whey)
Eggs,

Wheat
Barley
Rye
Millet
Oats
Gluten protein isolate
Soy protein isolate
Strawberries
Melons
Peanuts
Tree nuts
Fish
Seafood
Meat

You can check for food allergies and sensitivities yourself by keeping an accurate diet diary. Write down everything you eat and drink all day for three weeks. During that period of time make a note if you experience breathing changes, sores in your mouth, coughing, bloating, itching, or any other uncomfortable symptom. Look for an emerging pattern. Again, if you believe that you might have an allergy, stop consuming that particular food immediately!

Sensitivity to a chemical in your environment could also be the culprit. Look for chemical sensitivity in the same way that you would for a food irritant. This time you'll keep a diary of everywhere that you go to, and when you experience any symptoms. Tying the two together could identify the chemical that you're sensitive to. With chemicals, as with foods, don't be surprised if there's more than one.

It was a colleague of mine that first noticed I'd developed an allergy to nuts. One day she made the comment that every time I ate something with nuts in it I started to cough. Because coughing isn't something that I usually do, not even when I have a cold, this particular symptom stood out like a sore thumb. I didn't take the issue seriously at first. Not until the coughing began to lead into breathing difficulties. By process of elimination, I discovered that the primary culprit was the pecan nut.

I reiterate here that allergies can be dangerous. If you get hives, difficulty breathing, acute diarrhea or any other serious symptom, seek medical attention immediately. Allergies can quickly escalate into anaphylactic shock, which can be fatal!

I attribute the good health of my lungs to practicing Yoga Pranayama (moving energy with breathing exercises). If your issue with breathing is unrelated to a medical condition, allergies, or food or chemical sensitivity, then it's most likely due to being deconditioned. In this case I recommend practicing Pranayama for beginners. There's a segment on breathing under the heading 'MIND HOW YOU STRETCH'.

Taking a brisk walk is always a great way to start increasing your activity level. Walking outside is better for you both physically and psychologically. However, a treadmill is adequate if being outside just isn't possible. To find the correct pace for you, as you're walking repeat the following sentence, "I'm getting better every day in every way, and it's feeling really good!"

If you can say the sentence with ease, then you're walking too slowly. If it's a bit of a challenge to say but you can do it, you're at the correct pace. If you struggle to get the words out, and they trail off at the end, then you're pushing yourself too hard. This simple test is often used by personal trainers to determine your 'rate of exertion'.

If you need to carry items with you such as keys and a bottle of water, invest in a fanny pack or a small light backpack. You'll benefit more if your arms are freely swinging by your hips. This is a natural movement when walking, and helps to keep you balanced. Holding your arms close to your body, such as when holding a bag, uses more energy and detrimentally impacts your balance. Likewise, having something hanging from your shoulder can create muscle tension, and shift your center of gravity.

Being overweight can challenge your breathing, and make it difficult for you to increase your activity level. This can make it tempting to start skipping meals. Please don't skip meals in an effort to lose weight. Your body needs good quality food to give you energy. Many diet plans focus on counting calories, but in my opinion there's not enough emphasis on the quality of the calories being consumed.

Just because a gooey cake contains only one hundred calories, doesn't mean that cake will fuel the needs of your body. I personally don't read the number of calories on packages. Whenever possible I choose live unprocessed items. Nature knows best how to make foods that are complete and ready to eat. If you want to lose weight in a healthy way, perhaps you'd be wise to trust in nature too. Before you know it you'll be breathing a sigh of relief!

SEVEN: YOUR SPOUSE WANTS YOU TO LOOSE WEIGHT.

There are countless reasons why a person would do something just to please someone else. Kindness is high on the list of course, and is the most positive reason to please someone else. But duty is also up there on the list, along with feelings of guilt and obligation. When it comes to losing weight to please a spouse, the true intention is often obscured. The following are four ulterior motives that I've come across in my life coaching practice.

MOTIVE ONE: Playing a game of points.

Making lifestyle changes to please your spouse can be like playing a game of chess. You change your behavior to lose weight; this equates to you giving up your queen. Next you expect your spouse to give up one of his or her pieces to please you in return. Be clear about your motivation if you're going engage in this risky game. Playing tit-for-tat in your relationship is inevitably going to lead to a stalemate, and then nobody wins.

MOTIVE TWO: Believing that losing weight to improve one's appearance is vanity.

Losing weight to please your spouse relieves you of the stigma of vanity. Perhaps at some point in your upbringing the idea of confidence became mixed up with that of arrogance. This kind of confusion is inevitably going to knock your self-esteem. The purpose of making lifestyle changes is to improve your health, as well as your appearance. It's not healthy to feel ashamed of wanting to do something for yourself.

It may help to consider that your self-image is based on what you believe to be normal and acceptable. Thanks to movie stars, glossy magazines, and fashion models, what the average body should look like has been grossly distorted. Your body is uniquely yours, and is a reflection of your personal choices. There's no vanity in wanting to feel confident about the way that you look; in fact it's good for your health!

MOTIVE THREE: Trying to lose weight to please someone else averts responsibility.

Avoiding responsibility for your actions is a pattern of behavior, and won't be limited to just losing weight. When you set a goal to achieve something for yourself, you're in control of that venture. You're the one responsible for summoning the determination to succeed. If you fail there's no one to answer to but yourself. Trying to do something for someone else however, excuses you from responsibility should you fail.

If you're comfortable with your weight, but your partner isn't, then you have more important things to discuss than your diet. If you're not comfortable with your weight, then take responsibility for your body. Set your weight loss goals for yourself. Be determined to overcome all obstacles. You may be amazed at the response of your spouse to such a positive attitude. You may also be amazed at how good it feels to reach your goals for the sake of your own satisfaction.

MOTIVE FOUR: Losing weight to please a spouse may heal a failing relationship.

This reason is not only a recipe for failure of course, but an indication that there's a much more serious problem here. Changing your diet isn't going to heal a previous trauma. Losing weight won't improve communication between you and your partner. I'm not saying that losing weight is a bad thing for you to do. But if your motivation is to heal a failing relationship then it's a counselor that you need, not a dietician.

EIGHT: YOU'RE OVERWEIGHT AND FEELING EMBARRASSED ABOUT HOW YOU LOOK.

Feeling embarrassed is the result of self-judgment. Why else would you feel that you have something to hide from other people? Ironically it's your own standards that you're judging yourself by though. Just as you're comparing yourself to what you think is acceptable, you're also comparing other people that way. If you were sitting next an obese woman, do you think that she would have reason to feel embarrassed about herself?

Feeling the need to be approved of by others can be a powerful motivator; unfortunately it's not a positive one. Seeing yourself as unacceptable is just something that you've chosen to believe. Changing your physical body is only going to address the symptom; it won't eliminate the cause. This is particularly the case if the cause of your embarrassment is an underlying feeling of shame.

Feeling embarrassed about your appearance can begin in early childhood. Much of what you believe to be true you've learned from parents and teachers. If one or more of the educators in your life were critical of you, then you might consider this to be normal behavior and adopt it for yourself. Embarrassment and shame are learned behaviors that can be difficult to overcome, particularly when they're not recognized as such.

There's no need to delve into your past to overcome your feelings of embarrassment. There are so many positive reasons to achieve a healthy weight for your height and frame. Focus your attention on 'health improvement', rather than on losing weight. Choose to eat a healthier diet to boost your energy, so that you can enjoy all that life has to offer. Look in the mirror and admire the body that your new lifestyle is creating; there's nothing embarrassing about that at all.

NINE: IF YOU WERE SLIMMER AND HEALTHIER LOOKING YOU'D GET PROMOTED AT WORK.

Being told that you'd get a promotion if you lost weight may be a case for workplace discrimination. Being disrespected by a colleague because of your size creates a hostile work environment. Both of these situations could be remedied within the company. You can find out more about discrimination and harassment laws from the Human Resources Department.

There are going to be situations however, when it's not about the preference of a sleazy boss, or the ignorance of a coworker. There'll be times when the expectations are those of the society in which you live. A certain image is expected to be portrayed by people in certain positions. If you believe that you'd have more chance of getting promoted if you were slimmer, then you understand those expectations.

Physical appearance can certainly impact promotional opportunities for fitness and beauty professionals, receptionists, and PR representatives. More than likely the boss will consider the image of the company over the work performance of the employee. Remember that a boss has to justify his or her decisions, and face the consequences of them too. If your situations were reversed would you promote someone against your better judgment, and risk your own position within the company?

Making changes to improve your health, and to help you to clinch that promotion is a win-win situation. It won't be the only factor of course, but what do you have to lose other than that excess weight? Your determination to improve your health may well be enough to attract the attention of the boss. After that you'll need to be in tip-top condition to climb that corporate ladder!

TEN: YOU WANT TO BE A GOOD EXAMPLE TO YOUR CHILDREN.

I spent many summer evenings with my dad on the garden allotment [of land] at the back of our village house. Dad grew most of the vegetables for the family dinner in that garden. He'd pull up a handful of carrots and shake off the dirt. Then he'd pick out a full cabbage and drop them off in the kitchen for dinner. Many families were fortunate back then to live in small communities, growing their own food and bartering with other people.

Food was not labeled as 'organic' back in the days of my childhood. Most produce was grown locally and was automatically 'organic'. Food was eaten fresh throughout the spring and summer. Mothers spent their autumn days canning and pickling vegetables ready for the winter. Blackberry jam took the place of freshly baked blackberry pie. All remaining potatoes and onions were packed into mum's old stockings, and hung up in the shed.

Society today is more focused on cutting costs through mass production, than on good health and common sense. Our parents didn't need a degree in nutrition to create balanced meals. They ate what kept them healthy, and avoided that which didn't. Is it progress to feed children cheese burgers, greasy pizza, and chicken in a bucket - just because it's 'fast'? Do you really need research to show that poor quality foods are behind the health crisis today?

Your children are learning about how and what to eat from your example. They're also building their bodies using the fuel that you're providing for them. The bones in your son's body need quality food to create healthy new cells for growth. Your daughter's immune system needs balanced nutrition to protect her, and keep her well. Your own body is also re-creating itself every day, using the food that you're consuming.

Instructing your children to observe the old adage, "do what I say, not what I do" can't replace being a good example. Your offspring will learn what's good for them based on what they see you eating. How can they learn to eat whole grains and fruits for breakfast, when they see you chomping down on donuts, or pancakes and sausages? Being a good example to your children only requires that they see you being good to yourself.

ELEVEN: YOU'VE HEARD ABOUT GMO (GENETICALLY MODIFIED ORGANISMS), AND YOU DON'T WANT THIS IN YOUR FOOD.

Mother Nature has been genetically creating organisms for millennia, and doing so with perfect balance and sustainability. 'Modified' genetics are not the only problem that can be credited to mortals messing in Mother's business. Old growth forests are being decimated to grow crops. Rivers are being polluted with animal waste from factory farms. The quality of food has taken a dive, and the quantity consumed has rocketed in a vain attempt to compensate.

On a trip home to England one year, I went to visit a working farm that was open to the public. One of the barns had been set up as a picture room. From the left side door as you circled around the room the pictures told a story. The story began with the cost of trimming the hedgerows that grew around the crop fields. To save money the farmers had decided to cut down the hedges, and to replace them with wooden fences.

For generations the hedges had been providing a home for a species of ladybird [ladybugs as they're called in the US]. These tiny bright red beetles had a veracious appetite for aphids. Unfortunately the aphids had an equally veracious appetite for the crops. Without the ladybirds to keep their numbers down, the aphids quickly became a huge problem for the farmers. It turned out to be more cost effective in the long run to put the hedgerows back, and allow nature to keep the balance!

The devastating results of messing with Mother Nature's design can be seen all over the world. The USDA (United States Department of Agriculture) imported Kudzu from China for the purpose of erosion control. Sadly Kudzu soon became known as 'The Vine that ate the South!' It sickened my heart when I first saw the results of Kudzu in the North Carolina Mountains. Rows of trees appeared to have vanished under a blanket of this aggressive, non-native competitor.

In some circumstances we can clearly see the results of messing with the natural order of things. But what of messing with the building blocks of life itself? On the surface it may not always be possible to see the damage that's being done. The disasters waiting to befall us may not be apparent in the beginning. If you want to avoid being a part of this particular experiment, I suggest shopping for foods that are specifically marked, "non-GMO".

You'll find this quote on the WebMD page Genetically Modified Foods (Biotech Foods) Pros and Cons, Feature Archive Article, 'Are Biotech Foods Safe to Eat?'

"The U.S. government's position: Genetically engineered crops are safe, resist disease better, and can provide much-needed food in starving nations.

The EU position: Keep it out. We prefer organic, which is much healthier. The risk of genetically modified foods to health and the environment outweigh the benefits. Only the multinational biotech companies will benefit, dominating the world food supply and squeezing out traditional farmers.

The U.S. is the largest producer of genetically modified crops."

Although this list is by no means complete, foods that are commonly genetically modified are:

>Corn
>
>Cotton
>
>Potatoes
>
>Rapeseed (Canola Oil)
>
>Rice
>
>Soy
>
>Sugar beets
>
>Sugar cane
>
>Sweet-Corn
>
>Tomatoes

Packaged foods including candy bars, baby food and frozen dinners can contain genetically modified products, unless they're labelled 'GMO free'. Products containing GMO can crop up in places that you'd least expect. The following is taken from an article by Healthy Eating Politics entitled, 'Genetically Modified Crops:

"[In addition,] **commercial milk** producers inject dairy cattle with recombinant Bovine Growth Hormone (rBGH) which is a genetically modified hormone created to increase each cow's milk production. This hormone is present in the milk that comes from these cows. Not only does it sicken the cows in great numbers, it is linked to cancer in human beings.

The Canadian Journal of Veterinary Research published a meta-analysis of the impact of rBGH on dairy cattle. Findings indicated a nearly 25% increase in the risk of clinical mastitis (infection of the cow's udder), a 40% reduction in fertility and 55% increased risk of developing clinical signs of lameness."

I enjoy a variety of foods in my daily diet, including some that are on the list of commonly being 'genetically modified'. You can bet your bottom dollar though that I only buy organic, and those that are clearly marked 'NON GMO'!

TWELVE: YOU'RE CONCERNED ABOUT HIGH CHOLESTEROL.

Cholesterol' is a household word in our society today. It's not a four letter word, nor is it a disease; yet thanks to the media it's often treated as if it's both! TV commercials urge you to talk to your doctor about this condition called 'high cholesterol'. Of course the true purpose of these advertisements is to promote pharmaceutical drugs; and they're being paid for by pharmaceutical companies.

There's an old saying that goes 'a little knowledge is a dangerous thing'. Misleading knowledge can be just as precarious, when it comes to the subject of cholesterol. You may already be familiar with what's called 'good' or 'HDL', and what's called 'bad' or 'LDL'. What you may not know is that your own liver produces the wax-like substance called cholesterol. This natural substance is vital for many of the functions of your body. The following are a few of the bodily functions that require cholesterol:

1. Formation of hormones and cell membranes
2. Conversion of sunshine into Vitamin D
3. Metabolism of fat soluble Vitamins
4. Insulation of nerve fibers
5. Bile production

The terms 'good' and 'bad' cholesterol are actually referring to HDL (High Density Lipoproteins or 'good'), and LDL (Low Density Lipoproteins or 'bad'). In the word 'Lipoproteins' the Lipo part means fat. It's the type of fat that determines whether it will be labeled good or bad. LDL is only bad for you when you have more in your bloodstream than your body needs for healthy function. By understanding the relationship between cholesterol and fat, you'll better understand how this natural product of your own body came to get such a bad rap.

In simplified terms this is how it works: Cholesterol is produced by the liver, and binds to molecules of saturated fat and proteins creating LDL. LDL is the delivery system that takes the cholesterol to where it's needed in the body. Cholesterol is like putty; it's used to fill in cracks in your arteries. Only a small amount is needed. The cholesterol that's then released when your cells die binds to mono or poly unsaturated fats, creating HDL. HDL carries the cholesterol back to the liver, where it's either broken down, or passes out of the body as waste.

When you eat a healthy balanced diet this natural process goes on behind the scenes without a hitch. Problems can occur when you don't really understand what a 'healthy balanced diet' consists of. The following seven points may help to clear this up for you:

1. Your body needs a small amount of saturated fat for optimum function, and is capable of producing its own LDL.
2. Eating foods that contain saturated fat stimulates the liver to produce more cholesterol.
3. The majority of foods containing saturated fat are animal products. Saturated fat can only be found in a small number of vegetable sources, such as coconut and palm oil.
4. Hydrogenated vegetable oils known as 'trans fat' are not naturally occurring, and also stimulate the production of cholesterol.
5. The only dietary cholesterol is found in animal products: meat, poultry, dairy, eggs, fish, and seafood. In other words, you're eating the cholesterol that another animal produced for its own use.
6. Non-hydrogenated vegetable oils such as olive, sunflower and safflower oils create HDL, the good cholesterol. It's beneficial to have a higher HDL to LDL ratio, because HDL carries the excess cholesterol back to the liver.
7. Your body only needs a small amount of 'good oil' to function at optimum health. Attempting to offset LDL by adding more vegetable oil to your diet is ill advised. To help

lower LDL, eliminate the dietary cholesterol and saturated fat in animal products.

I clipped the following quote from the article 'cholesterol and heart disease', on the website of Physician's Committee for Responsible Medicine:

"Since our bodies make plenty of cholesterol for our needs, we do not need to add any in our diet. Cholesterol is found in all foods that come from animals: red meat, poultry, fish, eggs, milk, cheese, yogurt, and every other meat and dairy product. Choosing lean cuts of meat is not enough; the cholesterol is mainly in the lean portion. Many people are surprised to learn that chicken contains as much cholesterol as beef. Every four-ounce serving of beef or chicken contains 100 milligrams of cholesterol. Also, most shellfish are very high in cholesterol. All animal products should be avoided for this reason. No foods from plants contain cholesterol."

Even if you've been told that your high cholesterol problem is due to genetics, it makes no sense to make a bad situation worse. If you're seriously concerned about your cholesterol level, particularly if it's already high, observe the following:

1. Use only vegetable oils (mono and poly unsaturated fats), and keep them to a minimum.
2. Eat only plant based foods, because they don't contain cholesterol and saturated fat.
3. Avoid processed foods that contain trans-fat (hydrogenated oils).

THIRTEEN: YOU'RE CONCERNED ABOUT OSTEOPOROSIS, AND THE HEALTH OF YOUR BONES.

Osteoporosis doesn't have any outward symptoms, which is why it's also known as 'the silent disease'. Although accurate tests can now be done to determine bone density, often a problem is still only discovered after a fracture has occurred. Because bones are made up of living growing cells, preventing or slowing down bone loss is the best place to start. Bone loss is exacerbated by consuming excess caffeine, salt, and acid-forming foods. The following are some of the minerals and vitamins required to maintain bone health:

Zinc
Calcium
Magnesium
Vitamin D
Vitamin K

As I mentioned earlier, calcium is not only a vital component of bones, it also controls the pH balance of the blood. When acidity causes the healthy levels of calcium in your blood to drop, your body will pull more of this mineral right out of your bones to restore the pH balance.

Along with millions of other people in the western world, I was raised to believe that milk from a cow "does a [human] body good", particularly the bones. This information was being promoted in commercials for dairy products; commercials being produced and paid for by the dairy industry. Current research now supports that dairy does not do a body good at all; in fact the contrary to this statement is true.

The healthiest way to increase calcium intake, is to increase your consumption of green foods and beans. This will provide you with all the necessary minerals and vitamins required for bone health. The body more readily absorbs the calcium found in plant foods, than it does the calcium that has been added to processed dairy products.

The fact sheet, 'Parents guide to building better bones' by PCRM, refers to two studies done on calcium consumption and bone health. The following quotes are from these studies:

"In a 12-year Harvard study of 78,000 women, those who got the most calcium from dairy products received no benefit and actually broke more bones than the women who got little or no calcium from dairy." American Journal of Public health: Am J Publ Health 1997;87:992-7.

"Similarly, a 1994 study of elderly men and women in Sydney, Australia, showed that those who consumed the most dairy products had double the hip fracture rate of those who consumed the least." Cumming RG, Klineberg RJ. Case-control study of risk factors for hip fractures in the elderly. *Am J Epidemiol.* 1994;139:493-503.

The reason for the study results can be explained by the experts on nutrition at PCRM. Despite the amount of calcium in dairy products, other compounds also found in dairy accelerate the loss of calcium from the bones. Dieticians and nutritionists are now being educated by the latest research information. For a healthy skeleton, plant-based foods are now being promoted over dairy products.

Beans, including soybeans, are an inexpensive food that's rich in healthy bone building minerals. Always look for non-GMO soybeans of course. The American Journal of Epidemiology has this to say about soybeans:

"A quarter cup of tofu per day can result in a thirty percent reduction in fracture risk." Singapore Chinese Health Study, AM. J Epidemol 2009; 170 (7): 901:909.

Observing the following every day could improve the lifelong health of your bones:

1. Don't add extra salt to your food.
2. Eat plenty of leafy greens and beans.
3. Cut down, or preferably eliminate caffeine.
4. Avoid heavily processed foods, white flour and sugar.
5. Take the stairs whenever possible instead of the elevator.

6. Jump or skip if you are physically able to do vigorous exercise.

7. Avoid meat, and all dairy products: milk, cream, cheese, yoghurt, whey and ice-cream.

8. Spend at least fifteen minutes outside in the sunshine, or add a vitamin D supplement to your diet.

If you really enjoy milk and yogurt then look for calcium fortified almond, soy, rice, or coconut milk products. The company 'Daiya' also makes a fabulous cheese alternative that actually melts. You'll find Daiya cheese not only at Health Food stores, but at many local grocery stores now in the 'health food' section. These plant based products are also naturally cholesterol free. Keep in mind that all processed foods are best kept to a minimum.

Consuming calcium alone is not enough to increase bone density. You'll also need to add 'weight bearing' and 'muscle strengthening' exercises against gravity. These types of exercises stress the ligaments that attach muscles to bones. This in turn sends a signal to the bones to pull in more calcium for strength. Although swimming and cycling are great ways to stay fit, they're not ideal for bone-building.

If you're physically fit and able, then dancing, jumping, climbing, and lifting weights would be great bone-building exercises for you. Lower-impact exercises would be brisk walking outdoors, on a treadmill or elliptical. Walking up stairs holding onto a hand rail might be suitable for you. Exercising with low weight dumbbells or resistance bands can help to build the bone density of your upper body.

Osteoporosis is a preventable disease, but what you don't know about it could already be hurting you. Don't wait for the symptoms to show up before you take action. Osteoporosis is called 'the silent disease' for good reason. It's never too late, or too early, to make healthy life-style changes that promote bone growth, and prevent bone loss.

Your skeleton supports your body, protects your internal organs, and stores your minerals. The fact of the matter is that without your bones you wouldn't be able to do anything at all!

FOURTEEN: YOU'RE CONCERNED ABOUT THE PLANET, AND YOU WANT TO DO WHAT YOU CAN TO SUPPORT SUSTAINABILITY.

Children play games without giving a thought to how their actions are impacting the planet. Unfortunately, there are many adults doing just the same thing. The adult game known as 'commerce' can impact the environment with ripple effects. The destruction of the rain forest is a perfect example. Not caring about the impact of these actions is playing a dangerous game for everyone on Earth.

An individual cannot change the direction of a corporation, right? If you believe this statement to be true, then think again. Commerce runs on a system called 'supply and demand'. The demand is being created by the choices of every single person who goes shopping. You have the power to protect your home planet every time you visit the store.

To protect the environment you need to be educated about your food sources. Oceans, rivers, and forests are being contaminated and decimated to bring you substandard food. Food production has become more about quantity than about quality. Companies consider making money a priority over your health and wellness. You have the power to change that. As Mahatma Gandhi so eloquently promoted, 'be the change you wish to see in the world'.

Much of the population still labors under the illusion that meat and dairy animals graze peacefully outside in fields. They imagine farmers still scooping up cow and sheep dung in buckets to fertilize their gardens. The general public is mostly unaware of how Factory Farming has taken over the 'production' of animal based food. The following is from NRDC (Natural Resources Defense Council):

"Giant livestock farms, which can house hundreds of thousands of pigs, chickens, or cows, produce vast amounts of waste -- often generating the waste equivalent of a small city. While a problem of this nature -- and scale -- sounds almost comical, pollution from livestock farms seriously threatens humans, fish and ecosystems."

Hundreds of thousands of animals are tightly packed into sheds in just one farm alone! What do you think they're doing with all that pee and poop? What they're doing is keeping the waste in lagoons. These aren't lagoons of sparkling water surrounded by palm trees. Oh no, these lagoons are stinking cesspits. Can you imagine the horrendous results of an accidental overflow from one of these pits? The NRDC reports:

"Huge open-air waste lagoons, often as big as several football fields, are prone to leaks and spills. In 1995 an eight-acre hog-waste lagoon in North Carolina burst, spilling 25 million gallons of manure into the New River. The spill killed about 10 million fish and closed 364,000 acres of coastal wetlands to shell-fishing."

Some of the animal waste is used as manure. To get rid of the volume being produced every day though, way too much manure is put on the crops for them to absorb. Some of it runs off into rivers and streams. According to NRDC, more than forty diseases can be submitted to humans through manure.

The environmental damage to our beautiful planet doesn't stop at just polluting our rivers. The waste from factory farms contains ammonia. This ammonia produces nitrogen that causes algae to bloom. This algae, that shouldn't be blooming at all, then use up all the oxygen in the area. This is a major cause of dead zones where nothing else can live.

This quote can be found at the Grace Communications Foundation: Sustainable Table [Food Program]:

"According to the USDA, 'as much as 15 percent of the nitrogen fertilizer applied to cropland in the Mississippi River

Basin makes its way to the Gulf of Mexico.' This pollution is one of the leading causes of the so-called Gulf "Dead Zone," an oxygen-deprived area as large as 8,000 square miles—almost the size of New Jersey—in which no fish can survive."

Eating chicken instead of 'red meat' isn't doing your bit to solve the health problems of the planet either. Chickens are confined by the millions in factory farms. These farms are producing tons of waste every day. Chicken flesh is meat; just like the flesh of every other animal being consumed. It contains saturated fat and cholesterol. Eating chicken contributes to the ongoing damage to the environment.

Factory Farming isn't the only threat to the welfare of Mother Earth. Forty percent of the packaged foods in supermarkets contain Palm Oil. Palm Oil is a major crop being produced in the Tripa Peat Forest of Sumatra. What you won't be finding soon in the Tripa Peat forest is the Sumatran Orangutan! The very existence of this species is being threatened by Palm oil production. According to the COP (Center for Orangutan Protection):

"Palm oil companies are without doubt the cause of so much deforestation and literally the genocide of orangutans. Whenever we can we expose what they do, help rescue any orangutans (usually babies – their mothers having been shot or slashed to death with a machete) and we help local villagers resist approaches from palm oil companies and loggers."

The rain forests are not only known as 'nature's medicine chests', they're also home to more diversity of life than anywhere else on Earth. If this isn't reason enough to save them, tropical rain forests also 'breathe in' carbon dioxide and 'breathe out' clean air. Clean air is essential for human life to exist on this planet. The Amazon rain forest in Brazil is being cut down for an even more ridiculous reason - to provide grazing for cattle! This is from GREENPEACE:

"Brazil is the 4th largest greenhouse gas emitter, and has the largest commercial cattle herd in the world. The Amazon is being cleared to graze the cattle, and Brazil plans to double its production of beef by 2018."

If you're truly concerned about your health, and the health of your home planet, then do something about it. Use the power of your shopping cart. Stop creating the demand for foods that cause animal waste pollution and unnecessary deforestation. The volume of fish being eaten in homes and restaurants today has created the demand for huge commercial fishing vessels. Small village fishermen are being forced out of business, and the oceans are being depleted of life.

If humans continue to abuse this planet, nature will find a way to bring us back into balance. This will happen in the form of what we call 'natural disasters'. If you truly desire to live in a blissful body on a healthy planet, then do the following:

1. Buy locally grown plant based foods.
2. Look for organic whenever you possibly can.
3. Eat fruits and vegetables that are in season.
4. Avoid foods that contain palm oil; use healthier olive oil or sunflower oil instead.
5. Realize that eating chicken and fish is not the answer to improving your health, or to sustainability for the planet.

FIFTEEN: YOU'RE CONCERNED ABOUT YOUR FOOD BEING ASSOCIATED WITH VIOLENCE.

Even though I was born a decade after the end of World War II, people in the village where still talking about the death and destruction of it. Violence on such a massive scale leaves an imprint upon society. Events that would have shaken the village to its core prior to the war, paled in comparison to what happened in the trenches. People were no longer so easily shocked.

An event as dramatic as a war desensitizes people to violence. This then opens the door to acts of violence becoming commonplace and perfectly acceptable. Today, fighting and destruction is overt in movies, in the media, and even in games designed for children. Unfortunately, violence is also being consumed covertly in your food. This fact is well known by desensitized lawmakers. They justify their support of abject brutality by calling it commerce.

My first experience of killing didn't happen on the battle field. My first experience happened in the Butchers field in the village. The village junior school stood across the street from the Butchers. I remember a sheep named 'Lucy' being in the field at the back of the shop. In my memory Lucy had always been in that field. In reality, she'd probably only been there for a few weeks, or even days.

One day Lucy was gone. I remember finding out that she was in the butchers shop. Lucy was hanging up in pieces behind the counter.

Animals had been disappearing from that field long before I was born. Until that day I hadn't been old enough to understand what was happening to them. I can recall feeling differently about the Butchers shop after that event. I also recall though that no one else seemed to be affected at all by what had happened to Lucy.

Children weren't encouraged to talk about their feelings in those days. Things haven't changed much in some families today. Not that I would have known how to talk about it anyway. Just like other children all over the world, I was expected to accept what I was given to eat without question. I had no choice but to become desensitized to this socially acceptable violence.

The antonym for peace is 'war', and war is defined as violent conflict. A society that literally consumes violence every day is also desensitized to war. If this wasn't the case then wouldn't governments do everything within their power to avoid acts of violence? Unfortunately history demonstrates that violent conflict is not only acceptable, but often sought after and justified.

The civilization that created yoga understood the influence of diet upon their society. They observed the ramifications of violence, and chose to be vegetarians. Yoga practice began thousands of years before Europeans trampled their way across the Americas. The people that penned the ancient texts realized that a peaceful life is a life of compassion and respect. The first principle of the Eight Limbs of Yoga is Ahimsa. Ahimsa is a Sanskrit word meaning, 'non-violence in word, deed, or action to other beings'.

Mahatma Gandhi, a world renowned advocate for peace, recognized the benefits of practicing Ahimsa. He frequently used another Sanskrit word 'Satyaraha', meaning the practical implementation of non-violence. Gandhi realized the power of applying the principle of Ahimsa to every situation. From choosing non-violent resistance to British rule of India, to choosing plants over the slaughter of animals; Mahatma Gandhi was an enlightened teacher.

Sadly today, practicing Ahimsa has become 'compassion when it's convenient'. This can be witnessed in yoga studios all over the western world. Dedicated, caring, and spiritual 'Yogis' are as desensitized to the violence in their diet as every other unwitting citizen. Ahimsa has all but lost its deeper meaning. This empowering first principle is now thought of as little more than practicing random acts of kindness.

Given a choice, would you rather cut the head off a cabbage, or behead a cow? In society today you're no longer faced with such decisions about your food. You no longer have the obligation to truly 'feel' the ramifications of your dietary choices. If you had to experience what that animal, fish, or bird felt before its life was taken for you, would you still take it?

Albert Einstein is globally accepted as one of the greatest minds that ever existed. Dr. Einstein asserted in the following statement that desensitization to violence against animals cannot be beneficial:

"Although I have been prevented by outward circumstances from observing a strictly vegetarian diet, I have long been an adherent to the cause in principle. Besides agreeing with the aims of vegetarianism for aesthetic and moral reasons, it is my view that a vegetarian manner of living by its purely physical effect on the human temperament would most beneficially influence the lot of mankind." *Translation of letter to Hermann Huth, December 27, 1930, US (German-born) physicist (1879 - 1955)*

Albert Einstein made that statement over fifty years ago, when animals like Lucy the sheep still grazed in fields before their brutal end. Imagine what he'd say today about the billions of animals confined for their entire lives in cramped, windowless sheds.

Dr. Will Tuttle, author of the 'World Peace Diet', put it this way:

"By confining and killing animals for food, we have brought violence into our bodies and minds and disturbed the physical, emotional, mental, social, and spiritual dimensions of ourselves in deep and intractable ways.

Our meals [animal products] require us to eat like predators and thus to see ourselves as such, cultivating and justifying predatory behaviors and institutions that are the antithesis of the inclusiveness and kindness that accompany spiritual growth."

You react to violence, whether directly or indirectly, with fight-or-flight response. Your muscles tense, you breathe through your mouth, and you become hyper-aware of the danger in your environment. You may not be thinking about that pig as you tear the flesh off his ribs, but the knowledge of what you're doing is in your mind none-the-less. On some level, as a human being you know that it isn't natural or beneficial to eat another animal.

The groups that promote the consumption of animal products have always been aware of this fact. This is why when you go to the butchers you ask for a pound of beef, not a pound of cow's flesh. Pig meat is referred to as pork, and sheep as mutton. These animals have lost their identity as living beings altogether in our factory-fed society.

This desensitizing has sadly gone even further. When the correct names are being used for the animals, the animal is not the first thought that comes to your mind. What do you see when you hear the word 'chicken'? Do you see a plumb, glossy feathered bird pecking at the earth in the morning sun? Or do you see a lump of pale cooked flesh sitting on a plate?

I can't even say a lump of 'meat' in reference to chicken today. The poor chicken is no longer even recognized as having given up her meat for someone's dinner. The statement, "I don't eat meat anymore, just chicken and fish" is commonplace. What part of the chicken and the fish do you think is being eaten?

When you hear the words: lamb, ribs, and wings, what do you see in your mind's eye? Do you see animals and birds living out their lives in peace and freedom? More than likely you see a plate, a napkin, and a red and white bucket! This is the result of being desensitized to the violence in your food.

It may not be possible to live your life today completely free of aggression. It's absolutely possible to choose non-violence for yourself whenever you can. Mahatma Gandhi is attributed with saying, "Be the change you wish to see in the world". I can't think of any better words to live by. No one else has more power over what you experience in your life than you do.

If you don't want your food to be associated with violence, then choose what you eat wisely and consciously. The ancient Yogi's knew the secret, and they called it Ahimsa. A life lived choosing non-violence whenever possible is a life of compassion and caring. A life lived with the desire to resolve conflict, rather than to support it, is a life of peace and contentment. A peaceful life creates a blissful body. A life lived in a blissful body promotes a painless path.

CONCLUSION

The health care system is sadly lacking when it comes to the current chronic pain epidemic. Medical doctors diagnose symptoms, and prescribe medications; that's what they're trained to do. Surgeons cut, scrape, and sew, because that's what they're trained to do. Even Physical Therapists are limited to restoring function to a specific area of the body. Where does that leave the people who are suffering with symptoms that aren't related to an illness or injury? Where do you turn when the medications are dulling your life, as well as the pain?

Millions of people are dragging around chronic pain chains forged by everyday living. Their first link may have been the loss of a loved one, a job, or a relationship. That first twinge may have been felt after sitting hunched over a desk for years. No matter what the original causes may have been, the chains are getting heavier every day. Multitasking, demanding jobs, and destructive habits are adding link after link. Ironically, hitting the gym after a stressful day could be reinforcing a chronic pain chain, or could even be the start of one!

Sufferers of chronic pain can actually be their own worst enemy. The first hurdle that I often encounter is apathy. Apathy appears to me to be the result of our current cultural quick fix mentality. Why go to the effort of making lifestyle changes when a surgeon's knife could fix it quickly? There are times when a procedure is required to restore full function to a joint. An invasive surgery can have unexpected consequences though, and can ironically lead to more problems than you had to begin with.

In the past, having an operation required a hospital stay of several days, followed by a lengthy recovery. Today, surgery is frequently done on an outpatient basis. The disruption to your life is often little more than having a tooth pulled out. This doesn't necessarily make it the best option for your situation though. If you're in any doubt about needing an operation, get a second opinion. Educate yourself on all of the options available, including lifestyle changes as all or part of your program.

When surgery isn't an option at all, drugs are the alternative for many sufferers of chronic pain. Even over-the-counter drugs come with undesirable side effects. There's a time and place for muscle relaxers and pain medications. They're useful as a short-term support, but not as a lifelong crutch. In my own experience, medications only temporarily dull the experience of chronic pain anyway. Even the strongest drugs don't relieve the suffering altogether.

Pain is the language of your body telling you that something is wrong. Chronic pain is your nervous system stressing to get your attention. I've used my knowledge and experience in this book to help you to interpret the language of your body. The bottom line is that only you, the user, have the power to make lifestyle changes for yourself. Only you can overcome apathy, and form the good habits that will help to relieve your pain.

Habits in themselves have never been the evil enemy. Habits are patterns that you create to help you to efficiently use information. Problems arise when multi-tasking and juggling responsibilities lead to information overload. The pain signals from your body end up buried at the bottom of a long list of priorities. This leads to the second barrier that I'm often faced with overcoming: resistance to change.

Chronic pain that has plagued you for years could be relieved with something as simple as a correctly placed pillow. Yet knowing this is not necessarily enough to motivate change. Habits formed under stress are hard to replace. Stress puts you in survival mode, and the need to survive is a deeply rooted instinct. Your nervous system doesn't know the difference between a looming deadline, and a dangerous monster trying to kill you. Thankfully, you have the ability to become consciously aware of your self-destructive behavior, and to overcome your resistance to change.

Making the effort to break that chronic pain chain isn't just about your physical comfort and agility. Chronic pain disrupts your concentration, dampens your mood, and affects your enjoyment of life. Deliverance from the problem begins in your mind; first with knowledge, and then with awareness. Shedding light on your 'realization blind spots' leads you to the next step – taking action. Rearranging furniture, a new mattress, or better fitting shoes could put an end to your suffering. Finding relief from your chronic pain doesn't have to be hard work. On the contrary, living with pain is so much harder!

Self-awareness can be a tricky thing to achieve though. The habits that link your chain may not be as obvious as sleeping on a poorly sprung mattress. Your mental attitude can be just as hurtful, and more difficult to illuminate. Fortunately for you, there's a powerful tool at your disposal. This tool is called 'breathing'. Breathing is a bridge between your mind and your body. How you breathe speaks volumes about how you experience your life. Holding your breath, and breathing through your mouth are signs of flight-or-fight response. Huffing, sighing, and hyperventilating are all indications of what's going on in your thoughts.

Leaning how to breathe consciously could tumble down the walls of self-defense that you're suffering behind. Deep, slow breathing can appear to slow down time itself for you. Try it next time you're struggling in rush hour traffic. While you're sitting at that red light, focus on your breath. Make the outbreath slightly longer, and feel the weight of your body in the car seat. Now you've taken a little bit of knowledge, and used it to progress into awareness. Focusing on breathing is a way to live fully in the moment.

Try it right now. Take in a deep breath, and be aware of the weight of your body as you breathe out. Be aware of the tension in your muscles. Breathe in again, and consciously relax the tension as you breathe out. Let go of thoughts of the past, and worries of the future. Focus on your breath and be fully present. In just two or three minutes of your time you could be completely relaxing both your mind and your body.

Create mantas, affirmations, short catchy rhythms, or whatever you want to call them. Use them to anchor yourself in the current moment in a relaxed and positive way. For crazy traffic situations I created this one, "I am water flowing through the traffic on the path of least resistance."

Feeling chronic pain may be a normal experience for you, but it's far from natural. Likewise, aging doesn't have to be synonymous with stiffness, pain, and suffering. You're in your body for life - no send backs, no trade-ins. Stop making excuses to hold on to poor lifestyle habits; you're the only one that can make the necessary changes. Listen to what your body is trying to tell you. Now you know how to break the chains that are holding you down. You no longer have to imagine what it would feel like to find relief. You can enjoy living in a blissful body today!

BLISSFUL BODY - PAINLESS PATH

I free my thoughts from those that bind
I clear the clutter from my mind

I release myself from misery
Let peace and joy my feelings be

Let me go now chronic pain
That I might drop your heavy chain

I choose to live in glowing health
I choose to listen to myself

REFERENCES

Vivekananda Kendra Prakashan: YOGA: Asanas, Pranayama, Mudras, Kriyas: *BENEFITS [of Savasana].* 12th edition 1999, page 45. Published by Aye Yes Grafiks, Triplicane, Channai, India

NCCA (National Commission for Certification Agencies): www.credentialingexcellence.org

Splichal, Emily, DPM, Podiatrist and Human Movement Specialist at the Evidence Based Fitness Academy: *Training Specialist Certification*

Campbell, T. Colin, PhD: *The China Study*

Fuhrman, Joel, MD, http://www.drfuhrman.com: *FAQ: raw versus cooked*:

Dr. McDougall's Health and Medical Center: www.drmcdougall.com

American Heart Association: *High Protein Diets*, article January 3rd, 2012

American Diabetes Association, Fruits: http://www.diabetes.org/food-and-fitness/food/what-can-i-eat/making-healthy-food-choices/fruits.html

WebMD: Genetically Modified Foods (Biotech Foods) Pros and Cons Feature Archive Article: *Are Biotech Foods Safe to Eat?*

Healthy Eating Politics, www.healthyeatingpolitics.com: *Genetically Modified Crops.*

PCRM (Physician's Committee for Responsible Medicine) website article: *Cholesterol and Heart Disease*

PCRM referenced: American Journal of Public health, *Am J Publ Health* 1997;87:992-7, and Cumming RG, Klineberg RJ: *Case-control study of risk factors for hip fractures in the elderly. Am J Epidemiol.* 1994;139:493-503

American Journal of Epidemiology: *Singapore Chinese Health Study, AM. J Epidemol* 2009; 170 (7): 901:909

NRDC (Natural Resources Defense Council): www.nrdc.org/water/pollution/ffarms.asp

Grace Communications Foundation Sustainable Table (food program): www.sustainabletable.org

Center for Orangutan Protection: www.orangutanprotection.com

Greenpeace: www.greenpeace.org

Einstein, Albert (German physicist, 1879 to 1955): *Translation of letter from Albert Einstein to Hermann Huth*, December 27th, 1930

Tuttle, Will, PhD: *The World Peace Diet*